The Psychosis-Risk Syndrome

The Psychosis-Risk Syndrome

Handbook for Diagnosis and Follow-up

Thomas H. McGlashan, MD
Founder, PRIME Research Clinic
Professor, Department of Psychiatry
Connecticut Mental Health Center
Yale University School of Medicine
New Haven, CT

Barbara C. Walsh, PhD
Clinical Coordinator, PRIME Research Clinic
Research Associate, Department of Psychiatry
Connecticut Mental Health Center
Yale University School of Medicine
New Haven, CT

Scott W. Woods, MD
Director, PRIME Research Clinic
Professor, Department of Psychiatry
Connecticut Mental Health Center
Yale University School of Medicine
New Haven, CT

OXFORD
UNIVERSITY PRESS
2010

OXFORD
UNIVERSITY PRESS

Oxford University Press, Inc., publishes works that further
Oxford University's objective of excellence
in research, scholarship, and education.

Oxford New York
Auckland Cape Town Dar es Salaam Hong Kong Karachi
Kuala Lumpur Madrid Melbourne Mexico City Nairobi
New Delhi Shanghai Taipei Toronto

With offices in
Argentina Austria Brazil Chile Czech Republic France Greece
Guatemala Hungary Italy Japan Poland Portugal Singapore
South Korea Switzerland Thailand Turkey Ukraine Vietnam

Published by Oxford University Press, Inc.
198 Madison Avenue, New York, New York 10016

www.oup.com

Library of Congress Cataloging-in-Publication Data

McGlashan, Thomas H., 1941–
The psychosis-risk syndrome : handbook for diagnosis and follow-up/by
Thomas H. McGlashan, Barbara Walsh, Scott Woods.
p.; cm.
Includes bibliographical references and index.
ISBN 978-0-19-973331-6
1. Psychoses—Diagnosis. 2. Psychoses—Risk factors. 3. Diagnosis, Differential.
I. Walsh, Barbara, 1952– II. Woods, Scott, 1953– III. Title.
[DNLM: 1. Psychotic Disorders—diagnosis. 2. Diagnosis, Differential.
3. Interview, Psychological—methods. 4. Risk Factors. WM 200 M478p 2010]
RC512.M28 2010
616.89'075–dc22 2009045758

This book is dedicated in loving memory to
Tandy J. Miller, PhD,
who was Clinical Director of the PRIME Research Clinic from 1997 to 2005. She was a colleague, friend, mentor, and teacher whose wisdom and spirit live on in our hearts, our work, and the pages of this book.

Preface

At the Connecticut Mental Health Center in New Haven, the outpatient psychosis team of social workers, psychologists, and psychiatrists struggles daily with the Sisyphean task of keeping their chronically ill patients out in the community, on medication, away from street drugs, safe from the pit of homelessness, and, hopefully, relatively free from the daily terrors of psychotic realities. Such is the status quo of the "modern" treatment of schizophrenia.

From the perspective of the long-term institutions of the early twentieth century, the daily life of a person with schizophrenia has improved, but not by much. In the human nervous system, paralysis is paralysis, and that irreversibility holds for paralysis that is high up in the central nervous system producing psychosis, just as it does for paralysis at the level of the spinal cord producing paraplegia. However, a patient with paraplegia has an advantage over a patient with psychosis in that the paralysis is clear to everyone, making the wheelchair clearly necessary. For the psychotic patient, the underlying paralysis of capacities for perceiving, organizing, integrating, and communicating the "stuff" of daily experience is not immediately apparent, and the wheelchair of institutional support is routinely regarded as unnecessary and an infringement on one's civil liberties. As such, chronically ill psychotic patients bounce from one chaotic public shelter to another and from one emergency hospitalization to another.

What can be done? To begin to answer this question we must acknowledge that we do not currently have an answer, and proceed from there. One direction is to recognize irreversibility and to invest community resources in long-term support structures for the chronically ill victims of psychosis. Another direction is to explore the possibilities of preventing paralysis to begin with, which is why exploring the prodrome or risk-state to first psychosis has recently become of interest to mental health workers worldwide. This symptomatic and dysfunctional period leading up to the first psychotic "break" offers a new observational perspective into the neurobiological processes leading to psychosis. Furthermore, it offers a clinical syndrome to target for preventive identification and treatment.

The Structured Interview for Psychosis-Risk Syndromes (SIPS) is an interview and rating instrument designed to evaluate this clinical syndrome. It both generates diagnoses and rates symptom and syndrome severity. It is used to determine if a person was or is psychotic and, if not, whether that person currently meets commonly accepted criteria for being symptomatically at risk for becoming psychotic in the near future. Such symptomatic states are called psychosis-risk syndromes for first psychosis.

Because we do not know the etiology of psychosis we have no gold standard laboratory test to mark its presence. As such, at least for now, the diagnosis of psychosis relies entirely on manifest and/or reported symptoms, and therefore on symptoms that most people can observe and agree are present or not (known in the psychiatric diagnosis field as reliability).

The "official" diagnosis of psychosis in the American Psychiatric Association and International Classification of Diseases systems furthermore relies primarily on positive symptoms. Likewise, the identifying clinical features of risk syndromes in the SIPS are five positive symptom domains, specifically unusual thought content, suspiciousness, grandiosity, perceptual abnormalities, and disorganized communication. Why does the SIPS, like the DSM and ICD diagnostic systems for psychosis, rely so exclusively upon positive symptoms, especially since such symptoms are probably the last to emerge in the often lengthy process of developing psychosis? Positive symptoms are undoubtedly preceded in time by negative symptoms such as social anhedonia, amotivation, and functional deterioration. So why are these major "deficit phenomenologies" not the "diagnostic" symptoms? The answer lies not in any special link they have to the etiology of psychotic disorders. It lies quite pragmatically in the fact that positive symptoms have a higher signal value that something wrong is happening.

The later developing positive symptoms paradoxically are the underpinnings of early detection because even in their pre-psychotic form they are easier to see than the less visible negative phenomenologies and nonspecific symptoms of distress (anxiety, depression) that also occupy a place in the "psychosis-risk" realm. The disadvantage of positive symptoms being the diagnostic marker is that psychosis development is well underway when they emerge. The advantage is that prominent positive symptoms reduce the likelihood of making the mistake of saying someone is at risk when they really are not.

We, the authors, have used the SIPS at our psychosis-risk clinic in New Haven for more than a decade. We have also taught others at home and abroad about its application and utility. We attempt here, with this handbook, to condense and convey what we have learned about these syndromes of psychosis-risk and how to identify and describe them for clinical-research and, ultimately, for preventive treatment.

Since we do not yet have a laboratory test that can diagnose risk for psychosis, we are forced to rely on symptom observation to identify the risk syndrome in its later stages. It should not be forgotten, however, that earlier stages do exist, and efforts should always be made to characterize them with more precision. As such, the ultimate aim of the SIPS is to replace itself with a different set of criteria (including laboratory measures) that capture the clinical risk syndrome still earlier in the unfolding pathway to psychosis.

—Thomas McGlashan, Barbara Walsh, and Scott Woods
New Haven, CT

Contents

PART A

Psychosis-Risk Syndromes for First Psychosis: Background

This section introduces the concept of risk syndromes for psychosis and the recent history of efforts to identify its clinical and functional characteristics. Following this, our primary focus will turn to the rationale, development, and testing of one particular assessment system, the Structured Interview for Psychosis-Risk Syndromes (SIPS) and the Scale of Psychosis-Risk Symptoms (SOPS).

Chapter 1

Psychosis-Risk Syndromes for First Psychosis: A History of the Concept

The Prodrome: Earlier Terminology of Risk

The Psychosis-Risk Syndrome in the earlier psychiatric literature is often referred to as a risk state, or "the prodrome." The word "prodrome" comes from Greek *prodromos*, meaning the forerunner of an event. In the context of psychosis it often referred to the early signs, symptoms, and disabilities preceding the full onset of illness, i.e., a period of pre-psychotic disturbance that deviates from a person's typical thoughts, experiences, and behaviors.[1] The term, however, has also been used to denote early signs of relapse in persons who already have a psychotic illness and are in a remitted phase. Given this, and the fact that reference to risk states or periods is also common in other medical disorders (e.g., hepatitis), we will use "psychosis-risk syndrome" (for first psychosis) because of its greater clarity and specificity.

Rationale for Identifying the Psychosis-Risk Syndrome

Schizophrenia is a serious psychiatric disorder that erupts early during development and can be disabling for life.[2,3] It affects approximately 1%

of *any* population in the world.[4] The risk is somewhat higher for men, and the peak period of onset for men is 15–25 years of age and 25–35 years in women.[5] Onset in the teenage years is also common. This observation by Kraepelin in the early 1900s gave rise to the first name for schizophrenia—dementia praecox—or the dementing process that begins in adolescence.[6]

The costs of schizophrenia are enormous because the disorder disables early in life and its attendant deficits can last to old age, effectively robbing an entire adult life of productive capacity and requiring expensive treatment and remediation for the same period of time.[7] Treatments have improved from the days of long-term inpatient asylum care to the point where most patients can live in the community. At the same time, the majority of persons with schizophrenia remain symptomatic and struggle with deficits in self-care, work capacity, and interpersonal relationships[3] that too often are lifelong. Treatment can control most of the dangerous and disorganizing (positive) symptoms of the disorder (hallucinations, delusions, and disorganized thought, speech, and behavior), but their disruptive capacity is always a danger. They remain muted as residual symptoms and they can reactivate in the face of treatment noncompliance (which is epidemic to the disorder).

Given this status quo, the senior author of this handbook wrote as follows in 1996:

> I have had the pleasure of helping many patients with schizophrenia in my professional career and have seen clear advances in the understanding and treatment of the psychosis, so I remain optimistic. But my all too frequent encounters with the chronic and treatment-resistant patients of our work keep me focused on the half-empty part of the glass. I remain convinced with them I came upon the scene too late; most of the damage was already done. I remain convinced that with schizophrenia in its modest to severe form our current treatment efforts amount to palliation and damage control. There is no doubt that our efforts make a difference but they effect little if any restitution of what has been lost. For many vulnerable to schizophrenia, the ultimate answer lies in early detection and preventive intervention.[8]

There is also concern that many of the central nervous system neurobiological processes responsible for generating psychosis precede its onset by months or years and are irreversible by the time of onset.[9,10] As such, identifying psychosis in these beginning phases becomes an endeavor of paramount importance.

In order to think about early detection and intervention in psychosis, however, we must first become acquainted with the early stages of the disorder, what we feel drives these early stages, and the kinds of prevention that are possible to achieve.

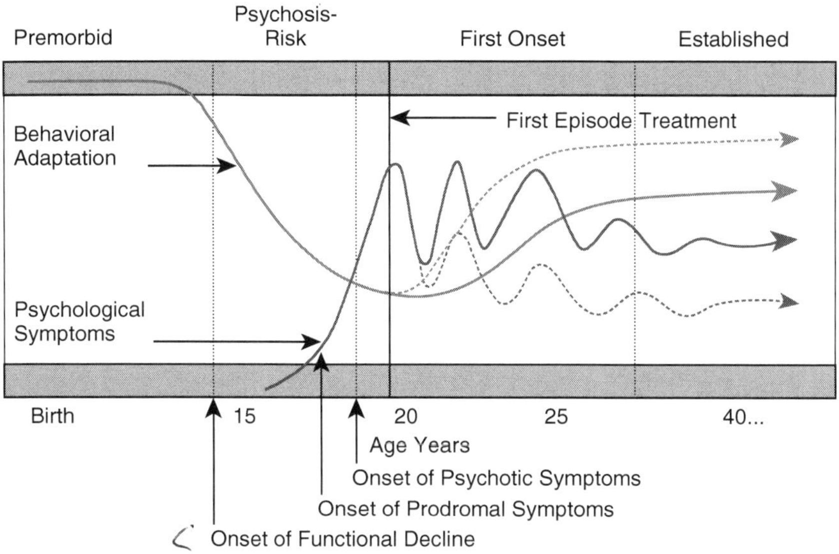

Figure 1.1 The early stages of psychosis.

The Early Stages of Schizophrenia

The early course of schizophrenia is schematized in Figure 1.1. It includes a premorbid phase, a prodromal phase, and a first psychosis phase.[11] The premorbid phase is a period of normality for most persons who ultimately develop schizophrenia. When deficits exist, they usually are manifest at birth and are subtle, stable, and usually not obvious or seriously disabling. In the second, or psychosis-risk phase, functioning declines in a clearly downward, usually accelerating trajectory. The psychosis-risk symptoms begin and develop with increasing number, severity, and frequency. The timing is usually around puberty. This phase lasts between two and five years on average.[12] The third, or first onset psychosis phase begins when “risk” symptoms become frankly psychotic, meaning persons feel convinced their hallucinations and delusions are real and they behave as if they are real. Insight and perspective are lost, and the capacity to function in an organized, integrated fashion becomes seriously compromised.

Neurobiological Processes Underlying the Development of Psychosis

Our model of the processes underlying the generation and onset of psychosis are detailed elsewhere[13] and schematized in Figure 1.2.

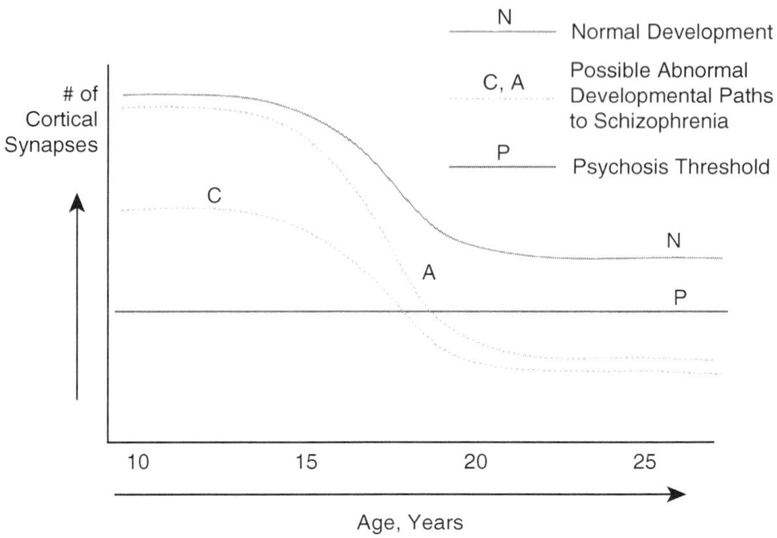

Figure 1.2 Model of developmentally reduced synaptic density/connectivity and the development of psychosis.
Based on McGlashan and Hoffman[13].

We consider the underlying course or pathophysiology of psychosis to be developmentally reduced synaptic density, or critically reduced connectivity, with a threshold schematized as line P in Figure 1.2. Below this line lies psychosis. Our model holds that in normal human development synaptic connectivity waxes and wanes according to phases of development. Synaptic connections normally blossom and multiply from birth to age five and then plateau until adolescence, when these connections are reduced or "pruned" to serve adult cognitive development. This normal process is seen as line N in Figure 1.2. The final adult brain has a reduced profusion of synapses but it possesses more efficiency as an overall computational entity.

Sometimes the childhood proliferation of synaptic connectivity is less than normal because of genetics, pregnancy and birth complications, etc. (see line C in Figure 1.2). The result here is less than normal brain synaptic density in childhood, sometimes manifest neurobiologically as deficits in social, academic, and/or cognitive functioning (the so-called premorbid deficits). For these children, normal adolescent pruning may be sufficient to reduce cortical synaptic reserves below the psychotic threshold (P).

In the other hypothesized pathway to psychosis, the childhood proliferation of synaptic connectivity is normally robust, but the pathogenic potential for psychosis lies in an abnormally intensified rate of synaptic pruning during adolescence/young adulthood. This is depicted as line A in

Figure 1.2. The ultimate outcome of the A trajectory is similar to that of the C trajectory, but the pathways and timing to psychosis may be different. For the C trajectory, disabilities are usually already present, precede adolescent changes, and often provide premonitory signals of problems to come. For the A trajectory, no such warning signals exist because the picture up to (and often through) early adolescence is completely normal. No clue exists that problems are forthcoming, and when they arrive, literally "out of the blue," they are often ignored and denied until the psychosis threshold has been breached, at which point any advantages that might have accrued from early detection and treatment are lost.

This handbook describes an assessment system that is sensitive to cases that are representative of both the C and A trajectories of psychosis development. The majority, however, belong to Type A because they are the most common, and because they are also the most difficult to see coming and to identify.

Types of Prevention Possible with Early Detection and Intervention

Three types of prevention are possible for many medical problems and disorders, and psychosis or schizophrenia is no exception. They are primary, secondary, and tertiary prevention.

Primary prevention strives to decrease the actual rate of disorders and/or cases in a population (also known as incidence). Preventive interventions usually target the cause or etiology of the problem, and the intervention is applied to everyone in the population. It aims to prevent the problem or disorder from happening at all. Examples are fluoridation of water to prevent dental caries or mandating the use of seat belts in cars to prevent death and injury from automobile accidents. Primary prevention in schizophrenia is rare if it occurs at all. It is known, for example, that Dutch women who were pregnant during a Nazi-induced famine during World War II gave birth to children who had a very modest but statistically significant increase in the rate of developing schizophrenia, i.e., on the order of 2% as opposed to 1%.[14] Thus it can be said that avoiding famine during pregnancy provides primary prevention against famine-induced cases of schizophrenia.

Secondary prevention does not prevent the disorder from happening, but it aims to reduce the prevalence of the disorder, i.e., the length and degree to which the disorder is present and active. It can reduce "presence" by delaying onset and/or preventing or delaying relapse. Secondary prevention efforts do not target the entire population. Rather, persons who are at high risk for developing a disorder are identified and treated. A good example is hypercholesteremia. Those in the population with this disturbance are at very high risk for developing heart disease and they are treated with antilipid medication in order to reduce that risk. Intervention here targets risk in a risk-defined population in hopes of preventing disorder.

Tertiary prevention aims to reduce the severity of a disorder while it is present and active, i.e., to reduce morbidity, course progression, mortality, and what is called collateral damage or the associated misfortunes that accompany being ill. In psychosis this usually means encountering difficult if not traumatic and destructive experiences such as being brought to the hospital by police because of paranoid terrors and loss of insight, or alienating friends who have become frightened by one's strange and irrational new behaviors.

Evidence That Early Detection and Intervention Might Be Preventive

Clinical research over the past several decades offers hints that very early application of existing treatments for schizophrenia might improve prognosis or the natural course of disorder. At the time antipsychotic drug treatment was introduced as a treatment for schizophrenia (in the 1950s), people who received these drugs earlier did better over the long term.[15,16] Many studies have measured the length of time between the onset of psychosis and first treatment (usually antipsychotic drugs and/or hospitalization). This time period, called the duration of untreated psychosis (or DUP), has become an important concept and measure because many studies have shown that earlier treatment after onset (shorter DUP) is correlated significantly with better outcome. Two recent reviews of these studies have been conducted [17,18] and consolidate this observation.

The TIPS study in Norway and Denmark is the first project that has actually tried to change DUP.[19,20] TIPS is a Norwegian acronym meaning "early intervention in psychosis" (Tidlig Intervention i Psychose). The investigation has shown that DUP can be reduced in a healthcare district through intensive education campaigns targeting the general public, schools, and general practitioners with information about the signs and symptoms of first psychosis and its treatment. Furthermore, these patients, when identified earlier in their ailment, are less disabled by symptoms, are less likely to hurt themselves, and are better functioning than patients who are identified and treated later in the course of their "first break."[21–27]

Treatment studies of people who appear to be experiencing symptoms of psychosis risk and who receive treatment, usually in the form of counseling and antipsychotic drugs, show a positive effect seen as delayed (and possibly prevented) onset of psychosis.[28,29] This effect has also been reported using purely psychosocial treatments such as cognitive behavioral therapy.[30] The original pioneer in this field was the late Ian Falloon, who set up a service in a UK healthcare district to identify people symptomatically at risk for psychosis and to treat them with home-based family therapy. Over the years that this service/project was in place he reported that the number of new onset cases of psychosis dropped to nearly zero.[31]

Overall, it is already apparent that early detection and intervention in the first episode and in the phase of psychosis-risk can achieve tertiary prevention (e.g., reducing suicidality) and secondary prevention (e.g., delaying onset). Primary prevention, i.e., preventing disorder altogether, has not yet been demonstrated but remains a possibility.

Chapter 2

Development of the Structured Interview for Psychosis-Risk Syndromes (SIPS)

Psychosis-Risk Syndrome: History of Its Assessment

The earliest efforts to track pre-psychotic risk for psychosis were conducted in the United States, Germany, and Australia. Chapman and Chapman[32,33] at Wisconsin developed "psychosis proneness" scales and applied them to undergraduate students in college. Over the next 10 years they found that 5.5% of students scoring high on the Perceptual Aberration or Magical Ideation scales developed psychosis compared to 1.3% of the lower-scoring student controls. This difference, while statistically significant, had low predictive value. That is, the scale was not very good at identifying *which* of the students would develop psychosis.

Starting in the 1960s Huber and colleagues[34] described subtle, non-willed deviations in thinking, feeling, and perception that they termed *basic symptoms* and later operationalized and tested as predictors of psychosis in a sample of university health clinic outpatients suspected to be at risk for psychosis.[35] Approximately 50% developed psychosis over the next 10 years. Here prediction was more accurate than the Chapman scale over the same length of time.

Alison Yung and colleagues in Melbourne[36,37] articulated psychosis-risk criteria that predicted the development of psychosis in the *near* future,

Table 2.1 High-Risk Syndromes

Brief Intermittent Psychotic State (BIP) Psychotic symptoms emerging in the recent past that occur too briefly to meet official criteria for a diagnosis of psychosis.
Attenuated Positive Symptom State (APS) Non-psychotic pre-delusional unusual thoughts, pre-hallucinatory perceptual abnormalities, or pre-thought disordered speech organization.
Genetic Risk and Deterioration State (GRD) Genetic risk for psychosis (first-degree relative with a schizophrenia spectrum disorder and/or schizotypal personality disorder in proband) plus a recent loss of social and/or work capacity equivalent to a 30% drop in GAF score over the past year that is sustained for at least one month.

i.e., within one year. These criteria identified three high-risk symptomatic and dysfunctional syndromes and are summarized in Table 2.1. The syndromes are a mix of recent-onset functional decline plus genetic risk and/or recent onset of subthreshold psychotic symptoms and/or recent onset of threshold psychotic symptoms that are briefly evanescent but not sufficiently sustained to meet criteria for a psychotic *disorder*. Forty-one percent of a sample (N=49) of outpatients identified by these criteria converted to psychosis within the ensuing year.[38]

The Pre-Onset Course of Schizophrenia and Predicting Psychosis

As introduced in Chapter 1, the early course of schizophrenia includes a premorbid stage, a prodromal or risk(+) stage, and a first episode psychotic stage of illness (see Figure 1.1, page 5). The premorbid phase refers to an asymptomatic period that may, in a minority of cases, include subtle and stable "neurodevelopmental" deficits in motor, social, and/or intellectual functioning. Such deficits appear at the time to be normal variations and usually mark a vulnerability to developing psychosis only in retrospect. Prospectively, however, such "risk markers" of the premorbid phase are mild and/or subtle at best and possess little, if any, positive predictive value (PPV) for psychosis.[39] PPV for psychosis is the percent of persons in any sample meeting risk marker criteria who actually go on to develop psychosis.

As detailed in Chapter 1 and illustrated in Figure 1.2, it is hypothesized that developmental changes, especially those associated with adolescence, initiate or accelerate neurobiological processes (e.g., cortical synaptic pruning) that go awry and become expressed psychologically as changes of mental, social, and instrumental functioning capacity, i.e., the risk phase of psychotic disorder. The majority of cases follow the abnormal developmental track labeled A in Figure 1.2. Clinically, this is expressed as a new and unexpected change from a person's normal, usual thinking, feeling, and behavior. If psychological/adaptive problems already exist (track C), they become clearly worse. The signal event in either case is a *recent change*, and the presence of such an event is the centerpiece of the SIPS psychosis-risk evaluation.

The first signs of disorder are usually functional, not symptomatic, and consist of newly appearing or newly accelerating *deficits* in social and intellectual functioning and organizational abilities. These changes, even though subtle at first, carry substantial PPV for psychosis. For example, over 42% in a sample of 16- and 17-year-old Israeli army recruits positive for such markers ultimately developed psychosis.[40] This represents an enormous gain in predictive power compared to behavioral and cognitive markers observed by teachers in genetically high risk and/or premorbid children from birth cohort studies, which typically have a PPV of only 5%.[41]

Psychosis-risk "symptoms" ultimately emerge alongside functional decline. Symptoms appear in 80%–90% of cases about six months to three years before the onset of psychosis. Nonspecific and negative symptoms usually develop first, followed by attenuated positive symptoms. In the year prior to onset, especially the last four to six months, symptoms accelerate in number and intensity. Their characteristic schizophrenic-like phenomenology (e.g., ideas of reference, paranoid ideation, unusual alien thoughts, unexplained sights and sounds) become more apparent, although elements of reality testing persist in the forms of doubt, skepticism, and disbelief. When these elements of insight become sufficiently attenuated, psychosis ensues.[42]

The Structured Interview for Psychosis-Risk Syndromes (The SIPS)

In 1997, McGlashan and colleagues developed an assessment instrument to rate psychosis-risk symptoms, the Scale of Prodromal Symptoms, or SOPS.[43,44] The instrument, renamed in 2009 as the Scale of Psychosis-Risk Symptoms, consists of scales to identify and measure five attenuated positive psychotic symptoms, six negative symptoms, four disorganization symptoms, and four general symptoms (see Table 2.2). All symptoms

Table 2.2 Scale of Psychosis-Risk Symptoms (SOPS)

SOPS positive (1–5)	1. Unusual thought content
	2. Suspiciousness
	3. Grandiosity
	4. Perceptual abnormalities
	5. Conceptual disorganization
SOPS negative (6–11)	6. Social isolation or withdrawal
	7. Avolition
	8. Decreased expression of emotion
	9. Decreased experience of emotion
	10. Decreased ideational richness
	11. Deterioration in role functioning
SOPS disorganization (12–15)	12. Odd behavior or appearance
	13. Bizarre thinking
	14. Trouble with focus and attention
	15. Impairment in personal hygiene
SOPS general (16–19)	16. Sleep disturbance
	17. Dysphoric mood
	18. Motor disturbance
	19. Impaired tolerance to stress

are rated on a scale from zero (not present) to 3 (present and moderate) to 5 (severe but not psychotic) to 6 (severe and psychotic) with anchoring criteria that are used to guide the symptom severity rating, detailed in Miller et al., 1999.[43] The scale defines severity variance in the subpsychotic or attenuated range, unlike existing scales such as the Brief Psychiatric Rating Scale,[45] the Positive and Negative Syndrome Scale,[46] and the Comprehensive Assessment of Symptoms and History[47] that rate severity largely in the psychotic range. The SOPS is embedded within a semi-structured interview, the Structured Interview for Psychosis-Risk Syndromes (SIPS), designed to diagnose risk syndromes according to the Chapter 1 criteria and to rate severity of the risk symptoms according to the SOPS. The operational definitions of these risk syndromes using the SIPS and SOPS are detailed later in Section B.

The SOPS and the SIPS were developed to accomplish three tasks: (1) to define the presence/absence of one or more of the three psychosis-risk states as articulated by Yung and colleagues (Table 2.1), (2) to measure the severity of risk symptoms cross-sectionally and longitudinally, and (3) to define the presence/absence of psychosis. In short, the SOPS and SIPS diagnose risk states, assess change in risk symptom severity, and diagnose when risk evolves or "converts" to psychosis.

Consistent with the DSM-IV definition of psychosis, the SIPS and SOPS define psychosis and two of the three risk syndromes using positive symptoms. The definition of a third risk syndrome rests not on positive symptoms but on family history of psychosis, a rating for Schizotypical Personality Disorder and the Global Assessment of Functioning (GAF) measure of functional capacity. All of these domains, as well as the SOPS, are incorporated into the SIPS interview.

Psychosis Threshold

Schizophrenic psychosis as defined in the DSM-IV[48] requires the presence of at least one positive "A" symptom of hallucinations, delusions, thought disorder, or bizarre behavior. Consistent with DSM-IV, the SOPS and SIPS define psychosis and two out of the three risk syndromes using the positive symptoms of Table 2.2. At the psychotic level of intensity, the five positive symptoms are delusions, paranoia, grandiosity, hallucinations, and disorganized speech. The corresponding five *attenuated* or *risk syndromal* positive symptoms are unusual thought content, suspiciousness, expansiveness, perceptual abnormalities, and discursive speech that is difficult to follow but not unintelligible.

The psychosis threshold scale in the SIPS is called the Presence of Psychosis Scale, or POPS. It, like DSM-IV, defines psychosis as the presence of at least one positive symptom at psychotic intensity for a "sufficient" length of time. The meaning of "sufficient," however, is not clear in DSM-IV. For DSM-IV Schizophrenia "sufficient" is defined as "a significant portion of time during a one month period," but what constitutes "a significant portion of time" is not further specified. For DSM-IV Schizophreniform Disorder, "sufficient" is an episode of disorder, including prodromal, active, and residual phases, that lasts at least one month but less than 6 months. Again, the period of time for active phase symptoms is not specified. For DSM-IV Brief Psychosis sufficient length is "at least one day but less than 1 month with full return to premorbid level." Time period is better specified, but is qualified by a retrospective judgment about remission. For DSM-IV Psychosis NOS sufficient length of active psychotic symptoms is not specified. In short, DSM-IV does not provide a clear or uniform threshold for the presence, and onset, of psychosis. Accordingly, for the POPS, we define psychosis threshold as the presence of at least one of the five positive symptoms at a psychotic level of intensity at sufficient frequency, duration, or urgency. Frequency/duration is operationalized as at least one hour a day at an average frequency of four days per week over one month, i.e., definite presence for more than half the days over one month. Urgency is any positive psychotic symptom that is "seriously disorganizing or dangerous" no matter what the duration.

Other dimensional scaling instruments of psychotic psychopathology such as the BPRS[45] or the PANSS,[46] measure the full range of severity of established, frankly psychotic symptoms. Not so the SOPS, which measures positive psychotic symptoms only to the threshold of psychotic intensity. Research protocols that must capture the full range of prodromal and psychotic intensities need to use the SOPS *and* a measure of psychosis such as the PANSS or BPRS.

An Alternative or Adjunctive Instrument to the SIPS and SOPS

Another psychosis-risk assessment system, the Comprehensive Assessment of At Risk Mental States, or CAARMS, is used commonly around the world for clinical and research purposes. It was developed by Alison Yung and colleagues at the PACE (risk syndrome) Clinic in Melbourne, Australia.[36]

The three types of psychosis-risk syndromes described above (attenuated positive symptom syndrome, brief intermittent psychotic symptom syndrome, and genetic risk and deterioration syndrome) were first articulated at the PACE Clinic, and the CAARMS was developed to identify which of these syndromal categories were met by persons being assessed there. The CAARMS in this context was crafted primarily to be a diagnostic instrument.

The SIPS/SOPS is also used to diagnose the PACE Clinic risk syndromes but in addition it defines and diagnoses a modified version of these risk syndromes. It is called the COPS or Criteria of Psychosis-risk Syndromes. The COPS syndrome criteria are virtually identical with the CAARMS syndrome criteria *except for timing*. The COPS requires that the positive psychosis-risk symptoms have begun or worsened in the recent past, e.g., the past year for the Attenuated Positive Symptom State (APS) and for the Genetic Risk and Deterioration State (GRD), and the past three months for the Brief Intermittent Psychotic State (BIPS). For the CAARMS, attenuated positive symptoms could have begun at any time in the past five years but need to be present in the past year.[49] They need not have worsened in the past year. A detailed comparison of the CAARMS and COPS can be found in Table 1, page 705 of Miller et al. (2003),[50] and will not be reproduced here.

To recapitulate, the CAARMS was originally crafted to be a diagnostic instrument. The SIPS on the other hand was designed to diagnose not only the risk syndromes but also the presence of or conversion to psychosis, and to rate the severity of risk symptoms longitudinally, i.e., to measure change with time and treatments.

Chapter 3

Reliability and Validity of the SIPS

Diagnosis and symptom rating scales in psychiatry must go beyond simply describing clinical phenomenology. They must describe symptoms and the diagnoses that are made up of different symptom clusters in ways that are reliable and valid. Reliability means quite simply that two different persons evaluating the same patient with the same rating instrument independently (i.e., without knowing the other person's ratings of the patient) agree on their ratings to a degree significantly better than chance. Good reliability is the most important "psychometric parameter" to achieve for any clinical rating scale, whether it be used for diagnosis or for monitoring symptom severity, because without it scientific counting, comparison, and hypothesis testing are impossible to achieve. Validity in risk syndrome clinical science means that groups of patients who are reliably assessed as being phenomenologically (e.g., symptomatically) distinct from one another actually prove to be distinct in ways that go beyond phenomenology, for example, in age range or gender ratio or family history of illness or severity of disorder or the level of long-term functional capacity.

The SIPS was first tested for reliability and validity in 1998, and the study is instructive about how these important psychometric parameters are generated. Patients were drawn from 81 consecutively recruited help-seeking individuals who gave written informed consent and were interviewed with the Structured Interview for Prodromal Syndromes from

January 23, 1998, through June 5, 2000. The patients had been referred to our psychosis-risk research clinic because of a suspected risk syndrome.

For the reliability study, 18 of the 81 help-seeking patients consented to videotaping of their interviews and they constituted the patient group for the reliability study. Their mean age was 19.6 years (SD=7.8), and 11 (61%) were male. In the reliability study, the original interview served as one rating for 16 of the 18 patients with complete data. All other ratings were made from videotapes.

The interviewers were trained in use of the SIPS through an apprenticeship model. Each interviewer must have previously co-rated four to five patients with one of the interview's developers and been judged by the developer as competent to administer the interview independently. A total of six interviewers participated as raters in the reliability study: one psychiatrist, one psychologist, three psychology postdoctoral fellows, and one research associate with extensive clinical experience (T.H.M., T.J.M., J.L.R., L.S., K.S., and P.J.M., respectively).

For each patient, the raters were blind to all other ratings for that patient although aware of the reason for referral. There were 58 ratings total, 3.2 ratings per patient, and 70 pairs of ratings. Kappa was computed as the reliability measure.

Of the 18 subjects in the reliability study, seven were categorized as risk(+) by the interviewer's assessment and 11 were categorized as risk(-)—of these 11, two were judged to be psychotic already with schizophrenia, and nine were neither risk(+) nor psychotic. The agreement among raters was 93% for the judgment of whether the subjects were risk(+) or risk(-), i.e., diagnostic reliability (kappa=0.81, 95% CI=0.55–0.93).

For the validity study, 35 of the 81 patients were ineligible; 29 entered a still-blinded clinical trial, four met the criteria for psychosis, and two were missing baseline data. Of the remaining 46, 29 (63%) participated in follow-up and constituted the study group for the validity study. Their mean age was 17.8 years (SD=6.1), and 19 (66%) were male. Of these 29, 13 met the criteria for a psychosis-risk syndrome at baseline, and 16 did not meet the criteria for either psychosis or the psychosis-risk syndrome. Of the 17 nonparticipants in the validity study, seven could not be located, nine refused to participate, and one was deceased. The mean age for these nonparticipants was 19.1 years (SD=6.3), 12 (71%) were male, and five (29%) had psychosis-risk syndromes; there were no significant differences between this group and the participants.

To track outcome, the Structured Interview for Psychosis–Risk Syndromes was conducted again at six and 12 months after baseline, and medication histories were reassessed. Most interviews were conducted face to face, but the interviews for four patients were conducted over the

Table 3.1 Six- and 12-month Outcomes of 29 Patients Evaluated for Psychosis-Risk Symptoms, by Baseline Status on the SOPS

Baseline diagnostic status	Number of Patients					
	6-month outcome[a,b]			12-month outcome[a,c]		
	Psychotic	Prodromal	Neither	Psychotic	Prodromal	Neither
Prodromal	6	5	2	7	4	2
Neither psychotic nor prodromal	0	0	16	0	2	14

[a] Psychotic outcome refers to schizophrenic psychosis. Significant relationship of diagnostic status at baseline to outcomes at 6 months and at 12 months (2x3 Fisher's exact tests, both $p<0.0001$).

[b] Significant relationship of diagnostic status at baseline to outcomes dichotomized as psychotic versus prodromal/neither ($p<0.004$) and as psychotic/prodromal versus neither ($p<0.0001$ (2x2 Fisher's exact tests).

[c] Significant relationship of diagnostic status at baseline to outcomes dichotomized as psychotic versus prodromal/neither ($p<0.002$) and as psychotic/prodromal versus neither ($p<0.0002$) (2x2 Fisher's exact tests).

telephone. At follow-up, patients initially categorized as risk(+) were diagnosed as still risk(+) unless they had developed psychosis or had remitted. The criteria for remission included the absence at follow-up of any positive symptom item in the Scale of Prodromal Symptoms with a score in the risk(+) range. Table 3.1 shows that six of the 13 baseline risk(+) patients (46%) developed schizophrenic psychosis by six months, and the rate was 54% at 12 months. Two patients' risk symptoms remitted. No patient who was initially not risk(+) developed schizophrenic psychosis, but two met the criteria for a risk syndrome 12 months later. This study clearly demonstrated that meeting SIPS criteria for a psychosis-risk syndrome placed the patient at significant risk for developing psychosis in the near future.

A more recent and much larger validity study of the SIPS was conducted collaboratively among eight participating academic clinical research centers spread across North America (Emory University, Harvard Medical School, UCLA, UCSD, University of North Carolina, University of Toronto, Yale University, and Zucker Hillside Hospital).[51] Each site recruited young persons who were help-seeking and who met psychosis-risk criteria as assessed by the same structured interview, the SIPS. Most raters in each site had been trained to reliability in using the SIPS by the developers of the instrument. As such, the individual site samples could be pooled to maximize sample size and generate high quality information about whether the SIPS was a valid predictor of new onset psychoses over the ensuing two and a half years.

Of the 370 risk(+) subjects enrolled in the study, 291 or 78.6% completed at least one follow-up. Of those 291, 82 had converted to psychosis over an average of two and a half years. Using survival curve analysis, the estimated rate of conversion to psychosis over that time if you met the risk syndrome criteria was 35%.[51] This represents a relative risk of 405 compared with the incident rate of all forms of psychosis in the general population during a comparable period of time.

Further evidence that the SIPS identified risk(+) groups are both unique psychiatric entities as well as high-risk clinical states was established by comparing this pooled NAPLS risk(+) sample to several groups such as normal controls (N=190), non-risk(+) help seekers (N=198), familial (genetic) high-risk subjects (N=40), and patients with schizotypal personality disorder (N=49). Comparisons were made on demography, symptom profile, functional capacity, comorbid diagnoses, family history of mental disorder, and follow-up outcome. Please consult reference 50 for details. Overall, however, the psychosis-risk sample proved to be more symptomatic than all groups other than Schizotypal Personality Disorder and to be at higher risk for conversion to psychosis over the next two and a half years than all of the comparison groups. These findings provide strong evidence of diagnostic validity of the risk syndrome for first psychosis.

Chapter 4

Symptom Classes and Factors in the SIPS

In medicine, symptoms are largely physical or "somatic" in their origin or expression (e.g., fever, rash, pain, paralysis). In psychiatry, symptoms are largely psychological and behavioral in their origin or expression. Examples of psychotic symptoms are hallucinations and delusions. Examples of behaviors seen frequently in psychosis include social isolation or impaired personal hygiene. Such behaviors are often referred to as symptomatic behaviors as opposed to symptoms proper, which refer to disorders of sense (e.g., seeing things that aren't there), disorders of judgment (e.g., seeing dangers that aren't there), disorders of ability to test reality (e.g., being convinced Martians are directing one's behavior via embedded transmitters), and disorders of communication (e.g., speaking unintelligibly).

The risk syndrome for psychosis, like psychosis itself, consists of symptoms and symptomatic behaviors. These are listed in Table 2.2 (page 13).

As can be seen, four types or classes of symptoms are listed: positive, negative, disorganized, and general. Positive symptoms include disorders of reality testing (delusions, persecutory ideas, grandiosity), of perception (hallucinations), and of communication (disorganized thinking and speech). They are called "positive" because they stand out as being new and strikingly different from "normal," i.e., thinking, feeling, and communication that is "unusual." Negative symptoms, as the adjective implies, refer to a diminution or an absence of normal "processes." These can include emotional and psychological processes such as drive, initiative, emotional responsiveness, and ideational richness, but they can also include behaviors such as self-care, social activity, and work. Both positive and negative symptoms are often alienating, i.e., they set persons apart from their group, their culture, even from their family. Disorganization symptoms include appearances and behaviors that do not "fit" with the person's social network and culture. Included here are strange ideas, odd dress (even for countercultures), rambling talk, poor empathy with others, and disheveled appearance.

General symptoms are problems common to many psychiatric illnesses, including non-psychotic mental illnesses such as depression or anxiety disorders. They can be regarded as representing nonspecific expressions of "illness" or "disability" and include problems with sleep; dysphoric moods such as distressing anxieties, fears, and depression; or an inability to tolerate and negotiate the stress of a "regular" day (e.g., the equivalent of someone with a fever requiring bed rest).

Symptom Factors

The symptoms listed in Table 2.2 have been sorted into four subscales based on similar descriptive phenomenology. Symptoms can also be "sorted" by the degree to which they occur together in actually affected patients. This is called factor analysis. Symptoms that cluster together to form a group of co-occurring symptoms are called factors.

A factor analysis was conducted on 94 subjects who met risk syndrome diagnostic criteria using the SIPS.[52] Their ratings on the Scale of Psychosis-Risk Symptoms measured the presence and severity of the symptoms listed in Table 2.2. These ratings were factor analyzed, and three factors emerged from the analysis. Table 4.1 lists all of the SOPS symptoms and the factors into which they aggregated. The three factors of this analysis are similar to our original discussion of the SOPS psychosis-risk symptoms clustering a priori into four subscales (Table 2.2).

All symptoms classified as **negative** within the SOPS load principally on **Factor 1**, along with "odd behavior or appearance" (SOPS-classified as a symptom of disorganization) and "conceptual disorganization"(SOPS-classified as a positive symptom). "Impairment in hygiene or social inattentiveness" also loads modestly on this factor, and not elsewhere. Symptoms loading on this factor are primarily negative in nature.

All four symptoms classified as **general** in the SOPS load on **Factor 2**, with three of them (sleep disturbance, dysphoric mood, and impaired stress tolerance) loading more heavily than the fourth (motor disturbances). A disorganization symptom, "trouble with focus and attention," loads

Table 4.1 Rotated Component Matrix of SOPS Items, Standardization Sample *(N=94)*

Symptom		Factor		
		1	2	3
D1.	Odd behavior or appearance	**0.74**		
N3.	Decreased expression of emotion	**0.71**		
N2.	Avolition	**0.62**		
N1.	Social isolation and withdrawal	**0.57**		
N5.	Decreased ideational richness	**0.53**		
P5.	Conceptual disorganization	**0.53**		
N4.	Decreased experience of emotionand self	**0.52**		
N6.	Deterioration in role functioning	**0.48**	0.38	
D4.	Impairment in personal hygiene and/or social attentiveness	**0.38**		
G2.	Dysphoric mood		**0.74**	
G1.	Sleep disturbances		**0.63**	0.47
G4.	Impaired tolerance to normal stress		**0.60**	
G3.	Motor disturbances		**0.39**	
D3.	Trouble with focus and attention		**0.60**	
P1.	Unusual thought content/delusional ideas			**0.78**
P4.	Perceptual abnormalities/hallucinations			**0.60**
P3.	Grandiosity		−0.41	**0.58**
D2.	Bizarre thinking	0.40		**0.56**
P2.	Suspiciousness/persecutory ideas			**0.42**

Extraction: Principal components analysis with varimax rotation.
Loadings <0.35 are not printed for clarity. Primary loadings are in **bold** typeface.

strongly on this factor, and "deterioration in role functioning," a negative symptom, shows a modest secondary loading. These symptoms are rather nonspecific in nature, and could reflect psychological disturbance or demoralization, perhaps in response to patients' recognition that they are experiencing disconcerting changes in functioning.

Factor 3 features primary loadings from four of the five SOPS **positive** symptoms, the exception being "conceptual disorganization" (Factor 1). "Bizarre thinking" (SOPS-classified as a disorganization symptom), also loads on this factor. "Sleep disturbance" shows a moderate secondary loading on this factor. Overall, this factor appears to reflect the positive symptom dimensions of psychosis vulnerability.

These symptoms and the clusters or factors into which they aggregate, both within individual risk(+) patients and within groups of risk(+) patients, are similar to those seen in the psychotic disorders (mostly schizophrenia) toward which many of these patients are evolving. The differences that mark these symptoms and factors as risk(+) as opposed to psychotic will be discussed next.

Chapter 5

Psychosis-Risk Syndromes and Psychosis in the SIPS

The psychosis-risk syndromes usually emerge "out of the blue" in the midst of the relative normality and quiescence of the premorbid period. One day nothing is apparent or amiss. A week or a month later something "is not quite right" and a new, more symptomatic and dysfunctional trajectory has emerged—the risk-syndrome. Insofar as we have only begun tracking this phase prospectively, our knowledge of its clinical features and their evolution to disorder remains preliminary. Nevertheless, a frequently observed trajectory starts with nonspecific psychiatric symptoms that become more clearly psychotic-like phenomenologically and evolve into one of three characteristic clusterings of symptoms and disabilities known as risk(+) syndromes. These syndromes, in turn, become more persistent and pervasive to the point where distress, disability, and an altered experience of reality become ascendant and ultimately lead to the appearance of, or conversion to, psychosis.

Clinical Features and Diagnostic Criteria

The natural history of the risk syndrome is characterized by nonspecific early symptoms of depression and anxiety followed by or concurrent with negative symptoms, including apathy, social withdrawal, and cognitive changes affecting concentration and attention. These symptoms are then succeeded by the positive symptoms of suspiciousness, ideas of reference, and perceptual abnormalities, which often serve as harbingers of the first episode.

Risk(+) patients as a group have several clinical characteristics in common. They (and their families) are aware of and distressed by their symptoms. The patients are both cognitively and functionally impaired. Their Global Assessment of Functioning (GAF) scale scores[53] are often less than 50 on a scale of 1–100, indicating serious symptoms.[50] These patients have often sought psychiatric treatment in the past and may have received psychotropic medications, including antipsychotics.[54]

The SOPS and SIPS of this handbook are used to diagnose the risk syndrome, to assess change systematically in risk psychopathology over time, and to identify psychosis. The diagnostic criteria for the three risk(+) syndromes and for psychosis are detailed in Table 5.1. In accordance with DSM-IV-TR, the SOPS and SIPS define psychosis and two of three risk(+) states by positive symptoms. The five positive psychotic symptoms are delusions, paranoia, grandiosity, hallucinations, and disorganized speech. The corresponding five risk(+) symptoms are unusual thought content,

Table 5.1 Diagnostic Criteria for Psychosis-Risk Syndromes and for Psychosis

	Diagnostic Criteria
Attenuated Positive Symptoms Syndrome APS	1. Abnormal unusual thought content, suspiciousness, and/or organization of communication that is below the threshold of frank psychosis. AND 2. These symptoms have begun or worsened in the past year. AND 3. These symptoms occur at least once per week for the last month. AND 4. Psychosis can be ruled out.
Brief Intermittent Psychosis Syndrome BIPS	1. Frankly psychotic unusual thought content, suspiciousness, grandiosity, perceptual abnormalities, and/or organization of communication. AND 2. These symptoms have begun in the past three months. AND 3. The symptoms occur currently at least several minutes per day at least once per month. AND 4. Psychosis can be ruled out.

Continued

Table 5.1. (continued)

	Diagnostic Criteria
Genetic Risk Plus Recent Deterioration GRD	1. First-degree relative with history of any psychotic disorder. OR 2. Schizotypal personality disorder in patient. AND 3. Substantial functional decline in the past year as measured by GAF. AND 4. Psychosis can be ruled out.
Psychosis	1. Frankly psychotic unusual thought content, suspiciousness, grandiosity, perceptual abnormalities, and/or organization of communication. AND 2. Symptoms are disorganizing or dangerous. OR 3. Symptoms occur more than one hour per day more than four times per week in the past month.

suspiciousness, expansiveness, perceptual abnormalities, and circumstantial speech that is difficult to follow but not incoherent. During the interview, a family psychiatric history, a rating of schizotypal personality disorder, and the GAF scale score are also obtained.

The diagnostic criteria for psychosis-risk syndromes in Table 5.1 describe three subgroups based on attenuated positive symptoms, brief psychotic symptoms, and genetic risk plus functional deterioration. In our experience, most risk(+) patients meet the attenuated positive symptoms criteria. A few meet the genetic risk plus functional deterioration criteria without meeting the criteria for attenuated positive symptoms. The brief intermittent psychotic symptom subtype appears to be rare.

Prototypic Psychosis-Risk Syndromes

The following disguised case vignettes from our PRIME Prodromal Research Clinic illustrate patients whose symptoms meet the criteria for one of the three psychosis-risk syndromes described above. Risk(+) patients can meet criteria for more than one syndrome simultaneously.

Case 1

Attenuated Positive Symptoms Syndrome

Angus, a single, 22-year-old Caucasian male, attended college full-time. He came from an intact family with no history of mental illness. For the past eight months he had become increasingly concerned about an image he sensed near him whenever he was in the bathroom of his apartment washing his face or showering. The image was that of a shadowy, vaguely female figure, whose presence was triggered by running water. He was frightened by the image and felt she was "spiteful" and wished that he would die by falling in the bathroom. Angus knew that it was not real, but it bothered him. He wanted treatment to eliminate the image and other images he reported first sensing in his childhood. The image appeared almost every time he entered the bathroom, so he avoided showering and washed only half his face at a time.

In his evaluation, Angus acknowledged that his friends regarded him as "weird" because of his preoccupation with themes such as the moral messages hidden in the music he played, the decline of civilization, and the special meanings he obtained from games of chess. He felt unmotivated, had subtle difficulty completing his homework despite maintaining a high grade point average, and procrastinated on his personal activities of daily living. He needed frequent prompts from his roommate to get up out of bed or go to class. He felt confusion once or twice a month, during which time he forgot what he was talking about in midsentence, and his friends noticed this. In fact, his girlfriend frequently complained to him that he was not the same.

Angus worried that other students wanted to exclude him from certain social groups and that he could overcome this by changing his hairstyle and his style of clothing in ways he could not explain. These concerns occurred approximately once every two weeks, and he believed that he was probably imagining them. He complained of feeling unmotivated and different from how he felt when he was younger.

Angus was judged to meet the attenuated positive symptoms criteria. The attenuated positive symptoms included perceptual abnormalities (sensing images in the room) and suspiciousness (people excluding him and talking negatively about him). The positive symptoms were considered attenuated rather than psychotic because Angus knew these experiences were not real even though they were clearly distressing.

Case 2

Brief Intermittent Psychotic Syndrome

Brian, a 16-year-old, African American high school sophomore, lived with his parents and older sister. There was no family history of psychotic illness. In the seventh grade, Brian became depressed and withdrawn and complained of difficulties concentrating and of problems with sleep. The parents attributed these problems to adjustment to junior high school, but the depressive symptoms resurfaced in his sophomore year.

During his initial evaluation, Brian was guarded and had constricted affect. He said that people at school disliked him and wanted to hurt him for reasons he could not specify. With detailed questioning, Brian admitted that he avoided two classmates because he thought he heard them calling him "a homo." He felt at the time that he was in danger of being assaulted by them but admitted that in retrospect they probably had not called him "a homo" or intended to attack him. However, he reported similar experiences with other classmates four to five times over the past three months, lasting only a few minutes and not leading to confrontation. Brian also had mild conceptual disorganization manifested as occasional circumstantial thinking but without other unusual thought content or grandiosity. His grades had slipped from mostly A's to mostly C's. His parents worried that if his performance continued to decline, he might have to repeat his sophomore year.

Brian was judged to meet the brief intermittent psychotic syndrome criteria. He had moments of paranoia that were of delusional intensity, but they were not acutely disorganizing or dangerous and were too brief to meet duration criteria for presence of psychosis.

Case 3

Genetic Risk and Functional Deterioration Prodromal Syndrome

Corine, a single, 19-year-old, Caucasian woman, worked at a fast-food restaurant and attended cosmetology classes part-time. She was the middle of three sisters, one of whom had been hospitalized for schizophrenia. Corine had felt depressed for at least a year prior to her referral and had been taking both a psychostimulant for ADHD and an antidepressant at various times with only moderate success. She reported trouble concentrating, had mismanaged her finances to the point that many checks had been returned for insufficient funds, and she was involved in chronic fights with her mother, which she regretted. One month prior to referral Corine thought she heard her name being called repetitively, and once in the month before her referral she thought she heard her compact disc player playing when it was turned off.

Corine was not motivated to do anything except spend time with her boyfriend and mostly she stayed alone in her room listening to music. She let leftover food accumulate on every surface in her bedroom. Corine was on the verge of being fired at work because of absenteeism, and she frequently did not attend beauty school. She complained of not having feelings when it was normal to have them. Corine was brought for evaluation by her parents, who expressed concern that she was showing symptoms similar to those they had seen before her older sister's first psychotic break.

Corine was a passive participant in the evaluation but endorsed depression and avolition. Although she acknowledged the concerns of her parents and promised to start engaging in more productive activities "tomorrow," the family noted that tomorrow never seemed to come. Corine said that she did not believe that hearing her name being called and hearing the compact disc player playing when it was turned off were real events. She said that these were "all in my head."

The number and strength of Corine's negative symptoms and her decrease in occupational, educational, and social functioning were dramatic. Her GAF scale score was judged to have declined at least 40 points in the past year. This functional decline plus the family history of schizophrenia in a first-degree relative satisfied the genetic risk and functional deterioration risk syndrome. Her positive symptoms were either too infrequent or too mild to meet APS or BIPS or Psychosis Criteria.

Prodrome Versus Psychosis

One of the key determinants of a symptom's being considered attenuated or prodromal and not at a fully psychotic level of intensity is the lack of conviction regarding the externally generated, "real" nature of the symptom as well as the maintenance of insight that a particular experience is, in fact, a symptom. For example, one high school student who was experiencing suspiciousness reported having the feeling that the entire freshman class in his high school was singling him out and watching him. He also reported realizing that this was not possible as soon as he checked on the gaze of one of his fellow students. Another young woman reported that even though she lived on the third floor of an apartment building in the city and knew that it was not possible for anyone to see directly into her window, she would sometimes feel that people were watching her and would sometimes not get undressed at night. One young man who reported grandiose unusual thought content reported that he had a "weird" feeling that if his coworkers brushed past him, they would have a better day. He was quick to counter, however, that he knew this was not possible.

Perceptual abnormalities in the attenuated realm can also be experienced at high level of severity that still fails to meet a psychotic level of intensity because insight is retained. Patients experiencing such symptoms can report hearing odd noises, such as banging or clicking or ringing, dogs barking when there is no animal present, or their name being called when no one is around. More severe but still attenuated symptoms have been described, such as hearing sounds or voices that seem far away or mumbled. Also reported frequently are vague perceptual changes such as seeing colors differently, seeing flashes of light, or seeing geometric shapes. People have also frequently reported noticing shadows out of the corner of their eyes or vague ghostlike figures.

Finally, because disordered thought is a subjective experience that is difficult for an observer to assess, the SIPS measures this experience through disorganized speech. Clinically, we look for people who over time have begun using odd words or unusual phrases, or who are beginning to have difficulty getting their point across, or who have become circumstantial or tangential in their speech. Circumstantial means speech that wanders in its theme but eventually gets back to the beginning topic or point. Tangential means speech that wanders and never gets back to the beginning.

Psychosis-Risk Versus Schizophrenia Spectrum Disorder (Schizotypy)

As captured by the three syndromes, the profile of risk for psychosis is considered to be a period of escalating severity of symptoms and/or functional decline that lies between the end of a relatively asymptomatic premorbid phase and the beginning of the frankly psychotic phase of schizophrenic psychosis.[54] The risk syndrome has some similarity on a conceptual basis to "spectrum" and other schizophrenia-related constructs but is sharply distinguished from them. The distinguishing features primarily relate to course and trajectory of illness. The risk syndrome construct is like schizotypy and schizotaxia in that symptoms are milder than in frank schizophrenia but it also differs from them in that symptoms are of relatively recent origin and escalating in severity rather than being stable and enduring. The risk syndrome construct is similar to the concept of genetic risk in sharing heightened risk for future progression to schizophrenia but differs in requiring that the state be symptomatic and in not requiring that family history of schizophrenia be present.

Risk Syndrome Versus DSM-IV Psychotic Disorders

The risk syndrome construct can also be compared and contrasted with DSM-IV conceptualizations of fully psychotic disorders that have not been present long enough to meet criteria for Schizophrenia proper or Schizoaffective Disorder (see Figure 5.1). These DSM-IV concepts are Psychotic Disorder Not Otherwise Specified (NOS), Brief Psychotic Disorder, and Schizophreniform Disorder. These DSM-IV concepts do not overlap with the APS or GRD or BIPS risk(+) syndromes. DSM-IV Schizophreniform Disorder mostly maps to definitions of full psychosis as operationalized either by the SIPS or by the CAARMS. However, as

<table>
<tr><td>Duration</td><td colspan="2">Days</td><td>Wks</td><td>Mos</td></tr>
<tr><td rowspan="2">SIPS</td><td colspan="4">SIPS Schizophrenic Psychosis
= an average of 4 days per week for 1 month
OR
= 1 day or less if symptoms seriously disorganizing or dangerous</td></tr>
<tr><td colspan="4">SIPS BIPS
< an average of 4 days per wk, < 3 mos
not seriously disorganizing or dangerous</td></tr>
<tr><td>DSM-IV</td><td colspan="2">Brief Psychotic Disorder
= 1 day but < 1 mo
Psychotic Disorder NOS
= 1 day, not yet 1 mo</td><td>Schizophreniform Disorder
= 1 mo but < 6 mos</td><td>Schizophrenia and
Schizoaffective Disorder
> 6 mos, including
prodrome</td></tr>
<tr><td>CAARMS</td><td>CAARMS BIPS
< 1 wk</td><td colspan="3">CAARMS Psychosis
> 1 wk</td></tr>
</table>

Note. BIPS = Brief Intermittent Psychotic Syndrome; BLIPS = Brief, Limited Intermittent Psychotic Symptom group; CAARMS = Comprehensive Assessment of At Risk Mental States; NOS = not otherwise specified; SIPS = Structured Interview for Psychosis-Risk Syndromes.

Figure 5.1 Relationship between duration of fully psychotic symptoms and diagnostic criteria for psychotic disorder and brief psychotic syndromes across 3 diagnostic systems.

shown in Figure 5.1, some patients who are late in the course of the BIPS risk syndrome as defined by the SIPS could simultaneously meet criteria for early DSM-IV Schizophreniform Disorder. For this overlap to occur, the brief intermittent psychotic symptoms would have to have been present between one and three months and also meet DSM-IV Schizophreniform Disorder criteria of being present "a significant portion of the time." Also as shown in Figure 5.1, a patient whose fully psychotic experience is of sufficiently short duration to meet DSM-IV criteria for psychotic disorder NOS or brief psychotic disorder could potentially meet either BIPS risk criteria or full psychosis criteria either using the SIPS or the CAARMS. Whether such patients meet risk syndrome or psychosis criteria for the SIPS depends on the duration or severity of psychotic symptoms, while for the CAARMS it depends solely on duration.

Chapter 6

The "Other" Symptoms of the Risk Syndromes: Negative, Disorganization, and General

As noted in Chapter 2, the positive symptoms diagnostic of the risk syndrome are often the last to develop. They are usually (in retrospect) preceded and/or accompanied by what are termed the "other" symptoms of the risk syndrome, negative, disorganization, and general. Negative "symptoms" are almost synonymous with losses of capacity and functioning, i.e., something is not present that should be present. General symptoms represent nonspecific markers of psychiatric distress such as anxiety, depression, insomnia, and poor coping with daily life. They are common but could be harbingers of several disorders other than the risk syndrome including depression, anxiety, post-traumatic stress disorder (PTSD), etc. Disorganization symptoms such as odd appearance, bizarre thinking, poor attention, or poor personal hygiene often identify someone who is in the residual or chronic phase of a psychotic disorder. However, such symptoms may also be seen in someone who is different, poorly organized, and compromised psychosocially even *before* the onset of the risk syndrome.

Negative symptoms are of particular interest because, at least theoretically, they may be the initial manifestation of the aberrant neurobiological developmental processes underlying the development of psychosis. They develop earlier, whereas positive symptoms develop later. The clinical manifestations of negative symptoms are best captured in Factor 1 of Table 4.1, especially the symptoms of decreased expression of emotion, avolition, social anhedonia, isolation and withdrawal, decreased ideational richness, and decreased experience of emotion and self.

Unfortunately, while negative symptoms may be an early sign of risk for psychosis, the symptoms themselves are often subtle and easy to overlook or explain away. They usually begin insidiously with a quiet loss of interests and a slowly progressive loss of capacities. Social isolation secondary to disinterest in others is very common. Spending more time alone doing less and less is also a frequent development. Such attitudes and behaviors are often misdiagnosed by parents and/or friends as normal, willful adolescent existential negativism. Only when it becomes extreme to the point of bizarreness and/or incapacity (e.g., spending hours in the bedroom literally doing *nothing*) does it become a signal of alarm, i.e., a symptom suggesting something amiss that is more than volitional.

By the time negative symptoms are recognized as such (if they are recognized at all), the psychotogenic process has usually progressed sufficiently that positive symptoms are likely to have begun. Positive symptoms signal more clearly that something isn't right. Unfortunately, however, they are usually kept private because they are new to the person, strange, and impossible to understand or explain. We find, for example, that it is often in the initial SIPS diagnostic interview that such symptoms are acknowledged for the first time.

Eventually the positive symptoms take the stage front and center because they alter perception, reasoning, and judgment in ways that have *high* signal value to family and community in the form of bizarre, irrational, and occasionally frightening behaviors that are very hard to ignore, deny, or explain away.

Because positive symptoms have such a high signal value, they form the backbone of the diagnosis of the risk syndrome just as they form the backbone of the diagnosis of schizophrenia. Yet it should always be kept in mind that these signals are *late* manifestations of a disease process that has already been underway for an unknown length of time. As such, negative symptoms are important to assess because they give clues as to how long the disorder underlying the positive symptoms has been active and developing, and as to how severe the disorder is likely to be in terms of chronicity and functional compromise.

Ultimately, the pathophysiologic processes that cause schizophrenia are likely to be the same as those that generate negative symptoms earlier and positive symptoms later, so future efforts at preventive early diagnosis and treatment will need to focus more on the negative symptom signals of disorder.

Scoring the "Other" Symptoms

Negative, disorganization, and general symptoms are rated on a 6-point SOPS scale like the positive symptoms, with one important difference. For positive symptoms, level 5 is labeled **Severe but not Psychotic** and level 6 is labeled **Severe and Psychotic**. For the "other" symptoms, 5 is labeled **Severe** and 6 is labeled **Extreme**. For these symptoms, no reference is made as to whether psychosis is absent or present. That decision depends solely on the positive symptoms, where a judgment of loss of reality-testing capacity can be made more clearly and reliably.

Chapter 7

Characteristics of SIPS Psychosis-Risk Samples

A large sample of treatment-seeking persons meeting the SIPS criteria for psychosis-risk was collected for a randomized clinical trial testing whether antipsychotic medication might delay or prevent clinical conversion from the prodrome to psychosis.[29] This sample of 60 persons was recruited over three and a half years across four sites in North America (Yale University, New Haven, Connecticut; University of Toronto, Toronto, Ontario; Calgary, Alberta; and University of North Carolina, Chapel Hill). The sample provides a first example of what the SIPS schizophrenia risk syndrome looks like demographically and clinically. It will be described in some detail below, understanding that further research and sample collection may add to or alter this profile.

The description will include what this group looked like demographically and diagnostically (its signs and symptoms), how the risk syndrome compares to other psychiatric disorders, how it can be differentiated from other disorders (differential diagnosis), and how common it appears to be in the population (epidemiology).

Measures

The measures used in this description are as follows. Psychosis-risk clinical status is assessed with the Scale of Psychosis-Risk Symptoms.[43,44]

Other psychopathology is assessed with the Positive and Negative Syndrome Scale,[46] the Clinical Global Impression–Severity of Illness Scale,[55] the Mania and Depression Rating Scale,[56] and the Young Mania Rating Scale.[57] Psychosocial functioning is assessed with the Global Assessment of Functioning Scale[53] and the Quality of Life Scale.[58] Premorbid functioning is rated with the Cannon-Spoor Premorbid Adjustment Scale.[59] Family history of mental illness is ascertained using the Modified Family History Research Diagnostic Criteria.[60]

Descriptive Characteristics (Demography)

The demographic details of the sample are shown in Table 7.1. The prototypic patient was adolescent, male, and single. The racial mix reflects the extant ethnic diversity of the four sites contributing to the sample.

Table 7.1 PRIME North America Psychosis-Risk Clinical Trial

Demography *(N=60)*		
Age		
Mean	17.8±4.8	
Median	16	
Range	12–36	
	N	%
Gender		
Male	39	65
Female	21	35
Ethnicity		
Caucasian	40	67
Hispanic	9	15
African American	6	10
Asian/Mixed	5	8
Marital Status		
Single	55	92
Married	2	3
Living with partner	3	5
Family History		
At least one first-degree relative with psychotic and/or affective disorder	27	45
Drug Treatment History		
Neuroleptic	7	12
Antidepressant	24	40
Anxiolytic	5	8
Anticonvulsant	2	3

A history of major psychotic or affective disorders in at least one first-degree relative was present in 26 study patients (44% of the sample). Within the affected relative group (not shown in table), schizophrenia spectrum psychotic disorders were the most common at 55%. Major depression (psychotic and non-psychotic) accounted for 45%, and bipolar disorder accounted for 7%. Diagnostic comorbidity resulted in a total percent greater than 100 due to overlap.

The majority of patients in this sample had been in some form of psychiatric contact prior to joining the clinical trial. Table 7.1 presents the frequency of prior psychiatric drug use in the sample. Antidepressants were the medications most frequently prescribed (40%).

The New Haven site accounted for the majority of the patients (N=39, 65%) followed by Toronto (N=9, 15%), North Carolina (N=6, 10%), and Calgary (N=6, 10%). A fifth site randomized one patient before withdrawing. The patient was added to the Calgary site for relevant analyses. Given that the enrollment period spanned 42 months (January 1998 to July 2001), recruitment efforts added approximately 1.4 patients per month to the protocol. At the New Haven site, for example, during the 42-month enrollment period, the PRIME Clinic received 476 phone calls, of which 162 were judged to be appropriate for a face-to-face evaluation. Of the 162 persons interviewed, 106 attended evaluation. Of this number, 61 or 64% were judged to meet COPS criteria for one or more of the three risk(+) syndromes. In turn, 49 consented to the study, and 39 ultimately progressed to randomization.

Diagnosis and Psychopathology

The overwhelming majority (N=57, 95%) of patients met criteria for the Attenuated Positive Symptom (APS) risk(+) state. Thirteen patients met criteria for the Genetic Risk and Deterioration State (GRD) risk(+) state, 10 of whom also met criteria for APS. No patient met criteria for Brief Intermittent Psychotic State (BIPS).

The frequency of risk(+) symptoms at baseline for the sample is outlined in Table 7.2. As detailed in the SIPS, positive symptoms were defined as risk(+) if the symptoms were rated between 3 (moderate) and 5 (severe but not psychotic) on the Scale of Psychosis-Risk Symptoms (SOPS). A rating of 6 indicated a psychotic, not an attenuated psychotic, level of severity. The most frequent positive psychosis-risk symptom was suspiciousness (60%) and the least frequent was grandiosity (17%).

As noted in Chapter 6, the negative, disorganization, and general SOPS symptom categories are not required for a psychosis-risk diagnosis but

Table 7.2 PRIME North America Psychosis-Risk Clinical Trial

Scale of Psychosis-Risk Symptoms (SOPS) *(N=60)*		
	N	%
Positive symptoms[a]		
Unusual thought content	29	48
Suspiciousness	36	60
Grandiosity	10	17
Perceptual abnormalities	30	50
Speech disorganization	29	48
Negative symptoms[b]		
Social isolation	47	78
Avolition	40	67
Decreased expression of emotion	25	42
Decreased experience of emotion	24	40
Decreased ideational richness	17	28
Decreased role functioning	46	77
Disorganization symptoms[b]		
Odd appearance	18	30
Bizarre thinking	19	32
Poor focus/attention	39	65
Poor hygiene	10	17
General symptoms[b]		
Sleep disturbance	22	37
Dysphoric mood	35	58
Motor disturbance	8	13
Decreased stress tolerance	28	47

[a] Number and percent of patients scoring between 3 (moderate) and 5 (severe but not psychotic)
[b] Number and percent of patients scoring between 3 (moderate) and 6 (extreme)

provide a measure of severity. A score of 6 therefore is labeled "Extreme" rather than "Severe and Psychotic." The frequency with which these symptoms scored between 3 (moderate) and 6 (extreme) are also noted in Table 7.2. The most frequent symptoms were social isolation (78%), decreased role functioning (77%), avolition (67%), poor focus and attention (65%), and dysphoric mood (58%). Substance use and abuse was present but infrequent, e.g., current use was absent in 93% of the sample for marijuana, 98% of the sample for alcohol, and 100% of the sample for sedatives, stimulants, cocaine, PCP, and opioids.

Baseline levels of psychopathology are summarized in Table 7.3. The PANSS-POS score is the mean of seven positive symptom criteria. Dividing the mean by the number of criteria provides an estimate of the average level of symptom severity for this cluster of symptoms. As noted

Table 7.3 PRIME North America Psychosis-Risk Clinical Trial

PRIME Sample Baseline Levels of Psychopathology *(N=60)*				
	N	Mean	S.D.	Average level of item severity
PANSS-POS	60	14.3	4.1	2.0
PANSS-NEG	60	17.4	5.9	2.5
PANSS-TOT	60	65.0	16.9	2.2
MADRS-TOT	60	13.3	8.7	1.3
YMS-TOT	60	4.5	4.1	0.4
CGI	60	3.7	0.9	
GAF-highest	60	57.3	12.8	
GAF-current	60	41.9	10.2	

PANSS: 2 = minimal; 3 = mild.
MADRS: 1 = questionable; 2 = mild.
YMS: 0 = absent; 1 = mild.
CGI: 3 = mildly ill; 4 = moderately ill.
GAF: 57 = a person with moderate symptoms and moderate difficulty in one area of social, work, or school functioning.
GAF: 42 = a person with some serious symptoms and impairment in functioning.

in the table, an average level of 2 corresponds to a PANSS severity level of "minimal." The average levels of severity for all of the PANSS symptom clusters (positive, negative, total) vary between minimal and mild. For depression (MADRS) the average symptom severity lies between questionable and mild, and for mania (YMRS) it lies between absent and mild. Overall, the average level of clinical severity as measured by the CGI lies between mildly and moderately ill.

In striking contrast to the relative absence or mildness of psychiatric symptoms on measures other than the SOPS, the level of functional disability as reflected in the current GAF scores is substantial. Equally noteworthy is the 15-point loss of functional capacity in the year prior to contacting the clinic (i.e., the difference between GAF Highest in the past year and GAF Current). This is a population that is clearly disabled despite a relative quiescence of symptomatic expression.

Premorbid adjustment as measured by the PAS includes estimates of several domains of functioning across four developmental levels, as noted in Table 7.4 which summarizes the scores for each domain at each level. Mild to moderate deterioration in adjustment over time and across developmental level appears to characterize all of the premorbid domains for this group. Between childhood and through adolescence, for example, social withdrawal increases, peer relationships drop away, academic performance suffers, and overall adjustment to school deteriorates. As noted

Table 7.4 PRIME North America Psychosis-Risk Clinical Trial

Premorbid Adjustment Scale												
Adjustment domain	Developmental level											
	Childhood (0–11 years)			Early adolescence (12–15 years)			Late adolescence (16–18 years)			Young adulthood (19 yrs and over)		
	N	Mean	S.D.	*N*	Mean	S.D.	*N*	Mean	S.D.	*N*	Mean	S.D.
Sociability and withdrawal 0=not withdrawn; 2=mild withdrawal; 4=moderate; 5=unrelated to others	54	1.8	1.7	55	2.3	1.6	33	2.8	1.8	17	2.7	1.7
Peer relationships 0=many friends; 2=close with a few; 4=relatives only; 6=isolated	54	1.8	1.5	55	2.3	1.5	33	2.5	1.5	17	2.9	1.6
Scholastic performance 0=excellent student; 2=good; 4=fair; 6=failing	54	2.2	1.6	55	3.7	1.6	33	3.8	2.0	—	—	—
Adaptation to school 0=good, enjoys; 2=fair; 4=poor, dislikes; 6=refuses school	34	1.3	1.2	55	2.2	1.6	33	2.8	1.8	—	—	—

in our discussion of negative symptoms, the prelude to positive symptoms in the prodrome is marked by insidiously accumulating failures at mastering the developmental milestones of adolescence and young adulthood. What emerges early are negative symptoms and failures to "thrive." While they are often a source of anguish for the patient and concern for the parents, they almost always are explained away as a temporary byproduct of "growing up." It is usually not until the positive symptoms begin that the psychopathologic nature of these early failures is recognized.

Other Psychopathology

While patients with schizophrenia are known frequently to meet criteria for co-occurring syndromes, diagnostic comorbidity during the developing (i.e., risk(+)) phase of illness remains relatively undescribed. However, several studies have begun to touch on the issue. In one published study, researchers found that help-seeking risk(+) patients had a rich history of contact with psychiatric services prior to their being identified as at-risk for emerging schizophrenia.[61] Other researchers have identified comorbid lifetime disorders,[62] comorbid baseline symptomatology,[38,63] comorbid substance use,[64] and comorbid outcome psychiatric diagnoses[65] among patients at high-risk for conversion to psychosis.

Rosen et al.[65] looked explicitly at comorbid psychopathology in help-seeking patients coming to a research psychosis-risk clinic, half of whom met criteria for being risk(+) (N=29) and half of whom did not (N=29). Patients in this study were evaluated for current and lifetime Axis I and Axis II psychiatric disorders using the Structured Clinical Interview for DSM-IV-Patient Edition (SCID-I/P)[66] and the Diagnostic Interview for Personality Disorders (DIPD-IV).[67] In an examination of symptomatology present at initial evaluation, 14 (48%) of the 29 risk(+) patients qualified for one or more current Axis I diagnoses (see Table 7.5). The most common current Axis I diagnoses were Cannabis Dependence and Major Depressive Disorder, followed by Alcohol Dependence. Twenty-eight percent (N=8) of the risk(+) subjects qualified for one or more current Affective Disorders, followed by 24% (N=7) with one or more Substance Use Disorders and 24% (N=7) with one or more Anxiety Disorders.

Results of this study indicate a frequent presence of both lifetime and current comorbid psychiatric syndromes in prospectively identified risk(+) patients. At the same time the presence of psychiatric comorbidity generally does not distinguish risk(+) patients from help-seeking control patients (indicating considerable overlap in clinical pictures).

Table 7.5 Current Axis I Diagnoses in Help-Seeking Risk(+) and Risk(−) Patients

Presenting Axis I diagnosis	Risk(+) (N=29)	Risk(−) (N=29)
Patients with one or more affective disorders	8* (28%)	7* (24%)
Depressive disorder NOS	2 (7%)	3 (10%)
Dysthymic disorder	1 (4%)	2 (7%)
Major depressive disorder	5 (17%)	3 (10%)
Patients with one or more anxiety disorders	7* (24%)	6* (21%)
Agoraphobia	1 (4%)	1 (4%)
Anxiety disorder NOS	0	1 (4%)
Generalized anxiety disorder	2 (7%)	2 (7%)
Obsessive-compulsive disorder	1 (4%)	0
Panic disorder	1 (4%)	2 (7%)
Post-traumatic stress disorder	1 (4%)	0
Social phobia	2 (4%)	3 (10%)
Patients with one or more substance use disorders	7* (24%)	4* (14%)
Alcohol abuse	2 (7%)	0
Alcohol dependence	4 (14%)	2 (7%)
Cannabis abuse	0	1 (4%)
Cannabis dependence	5 (17%)	0
Cocaine abuse	1 (4%)	0
Cocaine dependence	2 (7%)	0
Hallucinogen dependence	2 (7%)	0
Other abuse	1 (4%)	0
Polysubstance dependence	0	2 (7%)
Sedative/hypnotics/anxiolytics dependence	1 (4%)	0
Patients with adjustment disorders	0*	1* (4%)

All comparisons N.S., except cannabis dependence p = 0.052.

* As some patients meet criteria for one or more diagnoses, categories are not mutually e.

Epidemiology

The incidence of schizophrenia is approximately 1 new patient per year per 10,000 population, and the prevalence is 1% of the population worldwide. The gender distribution of schizophrenia is slightly higher for men. The most frequent period of onset of schizophrenia in males is the early 20s, for females the late 20s. Although meticulous epidemiological studies of the psychosis-risk syndrome have not yet been done, it is believed that the incidence of these patients will mirror that of patients with schizophrenia (approximately 1 per 10,000) but that the risk(+) patients will be on average one to two years younger. Recruitment efforts to date have been more successful with younger risk(+) patients, possibly explaining the tendency for a predominance of males in risk(+) samples because of their earlier age at onset. Finally, to the extent that current risk criteria cannot identify and eliminate false-positive cases, not all persons in psychosis-risk samples will develop schizophrenia. Until criteria become more specific, the risk syndrome will continue to include people who ultimately develop disorders other than schizophrenia as well as people who develop no disorder at all.

PART B

Psychosis-Risk Syndromes: SIPS and SOPS Evaluation

This section begins our focus on how to use the SIPS to diagnose the psychosis-risk syndrome and the SOPS to rate its severity. The instruments are designed for use by persons usually possessing at least a bachelor's degree who are trained to be clinicians or clinical researchers. Ideally the person also has experience using structured psychiatric interviews such as the SCID or PANSS. The examples used here come from our experiences in the PRIME Clinic in New Haven, Connecticut, at the Yale University School of Medicine. PRIME stands for Psychosis Risk Identification Management and Education, and the clinic has been in operation since 1996. Key personal details of all clinical examples have been altered to protect anonymity.

Chapter 8

Pathways to the Risk Syndrome Clinic

All persons who come to the PRIME Clinic are help-seeking. They are referred for a SIPS/SOPS evaluation from a variety of sources. Over its first 12 years of operation, the PRIME Clinic received referrals from the following sources: non-MD practicing clinicians in the community (33%), family members (22%), primary care and other MDs (20%), school-based personnel (13%), self-referral (10%), and other sources (2%).

Referrals are prompted by a variety of reasons and concerns. Parents worry about behaviors (usually new) that they see in their child such as not listening or following directions, doing poorly in school, or appearing not to care about others. Clinicians, on the other hand, report concerns about internal experiences that their patients are reporting. For example, a clinician may call seeking advice on a patient he or she has been working with for months. The clinician reports that he has been treating the patient for anxiety but recently noted changes in the presenting symptoms, e.g., that the patient had become mistrustful of others for the first time and had started experiencing some unusual thoughts that were new. The one constant for all referrals is that the patients have begun to experience worrisome changes in the past year that are in need of diagnostic clarification.

Phone Screen Interview (Appendix A)

The first contact is usually made by phone with the referring person (see Appendix A, the PRIME Clinic Phone Screen, pages 174–178). Review the screen in detail, then return to this text.

The purpose of the screen is to determine if a face-to-face SIPS interview is warranted. The SIPS/SOPS is designed to identify people who are at clinical high risk for a new onset of psychotic illness. For this reason it is important to ensure that there is a recent *onset* or *worsening* of symptoms and that the patient has *not* already been diagnosed or treated for a psychotic disorder or for any medical or psychiatric or substance-induced disorder that could account for the worrisome symptoms that prompted the contact.

Chapter 9

Initial Interview: The SIPS and SOPS Evaluation

The patient is soon to be in front of you, so it is the time to become acquainted with the SIPS (Appendix B, pages 179–236). Page 81 of the SIPS states the aims of the interview and details the criteria (POPS) used for ruling psychosis in or out. Pages 182–183 detail the criteria of the three psychosis-risk syndromes (COPS) for which the interview probes. Pages 184–186 provide instructions for rating the risk symptoms (SOPS). These rules and guidelines will be discussed at length in this chapter.

The initial interview or "overview" is outlined on page 187 with space for documentation on pages 187 and 188. This is followed by the Family History Grid (page 189), the Scale of Psychosis-Risk Symptoms (SOPS, pages 190–228), the Global Assessment of Functioning (GAF, pages 229–231), and the Schizotypal Personality Disorder checklist (page 232).

In the initial interview, if the patient is a minor, the interviewer should begin with the parent and child together to explain the interview process. Minors are always accompanied by a parent/guardian. In patients over 18 years of age, they may choose to bring their parent or perhaps another relative or friend to the interview.

Be sure to explain that the purpose of the evaluation is to determine a person's level of risk for developing serious mental illness and to determine if other conditions may be present. Explain that the interview is semi-structured and that the interviewer must ask every question; therefore, the patient may be able to relate to some questions and not to others. Let the patient know that his or her willingness to speak openly and honestly about his or her experiences will help to ensure that the evaluation will progress in a timely manner and will deliver accurate results.

Explain that after the background information and family history sections are completed, the rest of the interview will be conducted with the patient alone. When that section is completed, the interviewer will meet with the patient and family together to give feedback as to the risk determination for the patient. Inform everyone that the entire process may take anywhere from one and a half to three hours.

The purpose of the overview section of the SIPS is to obtain information about what has brought the person to the interview, recent functioning, and educational, developmental, medical, psychiatric, occupational, and social history. The overview should include: behaviors and symptoms obtained from the phone screen; occupational or academic functioning history including any recent changes; participation in special education programs; trauma history; developmental history; and medical history including medication, social history, and any recent changes; and history of substance use/experimentation. When the patient is a minor, it is particularly important to obtain the school performance and social/friendships histories when the parents are present and the substance use history when they are absent.

Past psychosis, if not ruled out via the phone screen, is evaluated at this time by eliciting information about past psychiatric symptoms, problems or treatments, including especially hospitalizations or treatments with antipsychotic medications.

Current psychosis is ruled out by using the Presence of Psychotic Symptoms (POPS) Criteria (see Appendix B, page 181 of the SIPS). Current psychosis is defined by the presence of Positive Symptoms at a severe and psychotic level for a long enough time. Ruling out a current psychosis requires asking about and rating the five Positive Symptom items outlined in the measure: Unusual Thought Content/Delusions, Suspiciousness, Grandiosity, Perceptual Abnormalities/Hallucinations, and Disorganized Speech. According to the operational criteria for determining the Presence of Psychosis (POPS) current psychosis is present (1) if a SOPS Positive Item is rated a 6 and the symptom is disorganizing or dangerous, or (2) if a SOPS Positive Item is rated a 6 and the symptom occurs for at least one hour per day at an average of four times per week over one month. An example of a 6 rating on perceptual abnormalities is a patient reporting that he hears the devil speaking to him and telling him to hurt himself. He believes the voice is real and he believes that he should act on the command.

This symptom meets criteria for being dangerous as well, and the patient would immediately meet criteria for current psychosis.

When determining the family history of mental illness, the interviewer should inquire about all first-degree relatives (i.e., parents, full siblings, half-siblings, children) of the patient. Be sure to document if the patient has any first-degree relatives with a psychotic disorder or other mental illness and their treatment history.

When discrepancies or conflicting information arise between patient and family, it is important to explore details with all parties present. Usually differences result from interpretations of the behaviors rather than the behaviors themselves. Nevertheless, unless the patient actually endorses specific symptoms and experiences, they are not recorded as present even if reported by family.

Collateral sources of information usually exist. If the patient endorses a symptom and a family member adds that he or she thinks it has been present for a certain period of time, the family member's assessment can be used for timing. Information from hospitals, doctors, and therapists should be considered valid even if denied by the patient. Prior hospitalizations are especially important to investigate since such an event may have been triggered by a psychotic episode. Whenever possible, copies of such records should be obtained, with patient/family consent of course.

Here is an example of the information obtained at the end of the first stage of an intake interview.

Dexter is a 14-year-old Caucasian male currently attending eighth grade at a local middle school. He lives with his biological mother and father and 15-year-old sister. He was referred by his psychiatrist for evaluation due to a recent increase in school-peer-related behavioral outbursts and anxieties as well as unusual thoughts and depression associated with these events. For example, when walking into the cafeteria he would notice his peers laughing and think they were laughing at him. He would then walk over to these peers and confront them with his suspicions in an intense, angry manner. He has been followed by his psychiatrist for four years but has had no hospitalizations or prescribed medications. The psychiatrist became concerned at this time because what initially appeared as anxiety or fear of rejection by his peers was becoming more of a delusional interpretation of events. This led the psychiatrist to make the referral. The patient reports no alcohol or substance use or experimentation.

His mother reports a normal pregnancy with good prenatal care. She reports no alcohol or other substance use during her pregnancy. The infant was born in good health and without any physical concerns. Developmental milestones were reached on time and there were no significant health matters during early childhood. The mother reports that the patient is quite intelligent and did very well academically in school. He began seeing his psychiatrist because of emotional outbursts in the school setting, which had a negative impact on his academic performance. He experienced a significant worsening of these outbursts four years later along with anxiety, depression, and an increase in unusual thoughts.

The patient's mother reports that she has a diagnosis of and is treated for a depressive disorder. She also reports that the patient's sister is diagnosed with dysthymic disorder.

In this case, no signs of psychosis were noted during the phone interview or in the overview section of the SIPS. It was therefore appropriate to proceed with the SOPS portion of the interview, asking the parents to sit in the waiting room while the evaluation was completed in privacy with the patient.

The SOPS is organized into four domains: Positive Symptoms, Negative Symptoms, General Symptoms, and Disorganization Symptoms. A risk-syndrome diagnosis is made based on the Positive Symptoms. Risk(+) range according to the COPS is a rating level of 3–5. Scoring a "recent onset" or worsening within this level puts someone into the range. The information obtained for the ratings in the additional domains provides both a descriptive and quantitative estimate of the diversity and severity of psychosis-risk symptoms.

All 19 items on the SOPS are scaled 0–6 (see SIPS, pages 184–186). Psychosis is defined by positive symptoms. To recapitulate, on the Positive Symptoms Scale 0 represents absent and 6 represents Severe and Psychotic. On the Negative Symptom Scale, Disorganization Symptom Scale, and General Symptom Scale, 0 represents absent and 6 represents extreme (*not* psychotic).

It is very important to ask every question in the "Inquiry" section of each item (see page 190). For any positive response to an inquiry, the interviewer should use qualifiers to obtain more detailed information. Inquiry is for lifetime although the time frame for rating current severity on each item is the past month.

Following each series of questions, a set of qualifiers is listed. Each question that elicits a positive response should be followed by these qualifiers in order to obtain more detailed information. The qualifier box includes the onset, duration, frequency, degree of distress, degree of interference with life, and the degree of conviction/meaning for each symptom, as well as the timing of the most recent significant increase.

Anchors in each scale are intended to provide guidelines and examples of signs for every symptom observed (see page 195). It is not necessary to meet every criterion in any one anchor to assign a particular rating. When in doubt about severity, revert to the headers of each scale level (i.e., questionable, mild, moderate, etc.). If you are still experiencing difficulty assigning a rating, then rate to extremes—specifically if score is between 1 and 2 then rate a 1, between 2 and 3 then rate a 2, between 3 and 4 then rate a 4. A rating of 5 is used for all severe positive symptoms without delusional conviction. Delusional conviction is used to distinguish a 5 from a 6 rating, which establishes a psychotic level of intensity. Queries used to make this assessment could include: How do you account for this experience? Do you ever feel that it could be in your head? Do you think this is real? Additional queries might include: Could this be your imagination? Does the voice sound as if it is "out loud" just as my voice is? Could someone else hear it?

The basis for ratings includes both patient reports and observed behaviors. Symptoms that are not endorsed by the patient after this process may not contribute to severity ratings. If there is a discrepancy in what is reported by the parent and patient, bring all parties into the interview room and discuss openly.

Each severity scale is followed by a "Rating based on:" section. After a rating is assigned, provide a description of the symptom(s) and the rationale for assigning the specific rating.

Following each "Rating based on:" section, four symptom qualifier boxes are filled out. A symptom onset box is listed. For positive symptoms currently rated at a level of 3 or higher, record the date when the earliest symptom first occurred at that level (i.e., "onset"). There is another box to record the most recent date when a symptom already rated at the risk(+) level scored an increase in intensity by at least one rating point. Different levels of symptom frequency are scored in the third box (the reasons for each are detailed later). In the final box a judgment is made as to whether the symptom reflects risk for psychosis or is more likely part of another psychiatric disorder. For Negative, Disorganization, and General Symptoms, an abbreviated symptom onset box is listed (e.g., pages 208–209).

The Positive Symptom Assessment

Unusual Thought Content (UTC) is the first symptom rated in the Positive Symptom domain (pages 194–195). This can be reported as confusion between what is real and imaginary, magical thinking, and ideas of reference. Ideas of reference are non-persecutory and therefore rated on UTC. Hearing your thoughts being said out loud so that other people can hear them is rated on UTC. Sensing a presence in the room is rated under UTC. It should be noted that there are times when a symptom may be double rated, depending on the presentation. For example, a patient may report that she often senses a presence in the kitchen of her house. The patient then describes feeling a pocket of cold air in the kitchen on many occasions.

Because this is a tactile sensation, this symptom would be rated on perceptual abnormalities. However, when asked how she accounts for this, the patient states that she thinks it might be the "ghost" of her deceased grandmother. This would then be rated on unusual thought content as well.

Let's return to Dexter and some of his unusual thought content. He stated that he spends an increasing amount of time thinking about different ideas and is becoming preoccupied with these ideas. He said that the time he spends thinking about his ideas has increased from 15% to 55% of the day over the last seven months. He feels that it is important to write these ideas down and to encode them in a private codebook. He carries the codebook with him, showed it to the interviewer and translated the title to the interviewer as "The Book of Ideas." It was written in hieroglyphic-like symbols that the patient said he invented. He also reported that when he reads the book at a later time, he occasionally finds his ideas trivial and cannot believe he needed to write them down.

In this case, Dexter is preoccupied with unusually valued ideas that are not easily dismissed. They are clearly compelling because they occupy about 55% of his day (i.e., the majority). Despite the fact that he later recognizes that these ideas are not profound, the symptom does not go away. This would rate a moderate (3) level of severity on the SOPS. Because it has begun or worsened within the past year and occurs on average at least once a week in the past month, it is diagnosable as being in the risk syndrome range.

The second positive symptom domain is Suspiciousness and Persecutory Ideas (pages 196–198). This includes the notion that people are hostile, thoughts of being watched or singled out, or the patient's behavioral display of a guarded or openly distrustful attitude. Hostile persecutory ideas of reference are rated here on suspiciousness.

Returning to the example of Dexter, he reported that whenever he walks through the halls at school he feels as though he has to be cautious so that nothing bad happens to him. He could not identify a person or persons who he thought might harm him, just a vague sense of feeling unsafe. It started at the beginning of the school year and was happening weekly. Dexter clearly has doubts about his safety and is sometimes hyper-vigilant despite there being no obvious source of danger. This would rate a mild (2) level of severity on the SOPS. This symptom has begun within the past year but because it does not make the 3–5 rating range it is not diagnosable as a risk symptom.

The third category in the Positive Symptom domain is Grandiosity (pages 198–200). This is an exaggerated self-opinion and unrealistic sense of superiority. There may be some expansiveness or boastfulness present. Dexter stated, "I don't mean to brag but I tend to think in a wide way, with variety and color—like in a worldly, mature way." He reported that he has excellent skills at computer games. He says he has the reading level of an 18-year-old and that he is planning to write a Tolkien-type book. [Email note to Barbara] He stated that he started feeling this way three months ago and it occurs nearly every day. Dexter is expansive, expressing the notion of being unusually gifted or special. This would rate a moderate (3) level of intensity on the SOPS rating scale. It began in the past year and occurs on average at least once a week over the past month, so it is diagnosable in the risk syndrome range.

Perceptual Abnormalities/Hallucinations is the fourth symptom in the Positive Symptom domain (pages 201–205). This could be represented by unusual perceptual experiences, heightened or dulled perceptions, vivid sensory experiences, distortions or illusions, or hearing your own thoughts as if they are being spoken outside of your head. Seeing ghostlike figures would also be rated here on perceptual abnormalities. Dexter stated that when he walks in the halls at school he hears his name being called even when no one is there. He said this occurs about three times per month. This experience has begun in the past year and he is uncertain what to make of it. He reported that when he hears his name being called he often turns to look to see if someone is really there or he asks someone else if they heard it too.

Dexter is reporting a persistent auditory perceptual distortion that is experienced as unusual and somewhat worrisome so that he does a reality check. This would rate a moderate (3) level of severity on the SOPS rating scale. This symptom has begun in the past year but has only occurred three times in the past month. Therefore, it is not diagnosable in the risk syndrome range because it does not meet the average frequency of once a week in the past month. It is important to note that a reality check does not constitute a change in behavior. In the above example, a change in behavior would be if Dexter avoided walking down certain corridors in school because of the experience.

Disorganized Communication is the final symptom in the Positive Symptom domain (pages 205–207). This is when the patient uses overelaborate speech, or is tangential or circumstantial. The patient could also communicate in a vague, confused, or muddled fashion.

Dexter stated that people sometimes tell him they cannot understand him when he speaks, and that he sometimes talks in circles. During the interview he rambled occasionally and required some redirection from the interviewer. He reported that this happens every day and has occurred ever since he began talking. It was not getting worse. Dexter exhibited wandering off track and into occasional irrelevant topics during the interview. He did respond to clarifying questions and redirection. This would rate at a moderate (3) level of severity on the SOPS Disorganized Communication rating scale. Due to the longstanding and stable nature of this symptom, however, it is not diagnosable in the risk(+) range.

Because Dexter reported symptoms of disorganized communication *and* exhibited them in the interview, this makes the rating very solid. When a patient reports symptoms of disorganized communication but no signs or symptoms are exhibited during the long interview, the interviewer would rate the symptom at a questionably present (1) level of severity.

At the end of the Positive Symptom domain ratings, it is clear that Dexter meets criteria for the Attenuated Positive Symptom Psychosis-Risk Syndrome. A person only needs to receive a score of 3–5 on one symptom in the positive symptom domain to meet risk criteria, as long as the symptom also began or worsened in the past year and meets frequency criteria. Dexter received a rating of 3 for items P1 and P3, and both of these symptoms began or worsened in the past year and occurred on average at least once a week over the past month.

Assessment of Remaining Prodromal Symptoms and Completing the SIPS Ratings

Even though we now know that Dexter meets criteria for a psychosis-risk syndrome, we continue the evaluation using the SOPS rating scales for Negative, Disorganization, and General Symptoms (Appendix B, pages 208–228). While this additional information will not contribute to the diagnosis of a risk syndrome, it will provide both a descriptive and a quantitative measure of the diversity and severity of risk symptoms.

It is important that the interviewer recognize that language and culture are important considerations when making the SOPS ratings. For example, proverbs in the Ideational Richness section may need to be adapted for each language/culture, and what is considered to be normative can vary from culture to culture.

The SOPS describes and rates psychosis-risk and other symptoms that have occurred in the past month (or since the last rating). The SOPS measures both severity and change. The SOPS final ratings are recorded on the summary sheet at the end of the SIPS (pages 235, 236).

Differential Diagnostic Assessment for Other Disorders That May Account for the Psychosis-Risk Symptoms

Many of the signs and symptoms we see and rate in the SIPS and SOPS can also be psychiatric signals of the presence of problems and disorders other than the risk syndrome for first psychosis. The nature of psychiatric disorders in general is that different disorders share many of the same psychological symptoms. Anxiety, for example, is experienced when a person begins to feel that he or she is being watched (risk for paranoia), but anxiety can also be an expression of a phobia such as a fear of the outside known as agoraphobia. Because of this, whenever the initial SIPS assessment suggests the presence of a risk for first psychosis, a comprehensive psychiatric assessment must then be made to rule out that the risk syndrome picture (and diagnosis) is not better accounted for by another psychiatric diagnosis.

This task is called establishing a differential diagnostic list of disorders that might better account for the "risk" signs and symptoms being endorsed by the patient under evaluation. Because the diagnosis of most psychiatric disorders is still based upon presenting psychiatric signs and symptoms, the differential diagnostic task must be comprehensive and can be time-consuming. In our clinic we do a general psychiatric evaluation of the patient for DSM-IV Axis I and Axis II disorders with one or another structured interview such as the SCID[66] (Structured Clinical Interview for DSM psychiatric disorders).

There are two tests for whether the possible risk symptoms are better accounted for by another DSM diagnosis. The first test is temporal sequence. If the symptoms persist when the co-occurring diagnosis in is remission or were present before onset of the co-occurring disorder, a risk syndrome diagnosis is given when all other criteria are met. If the co-occurring diagnosis has been present continuously during the period of otherwise qualifying symptoms, the second test is applied.

The second test is whether the attenuated positive symptoms are more characteristic of a risk syndrome or more characteristic of the co-occurring disorder. When the symptoms are more characteristic of the other disorder, the symptoms are considered better accounted for by the other disorder, and a risk syndrome diagnosis is not given.

When such an assessment is finished, and the presence of one or more psychiatric disorders has been established, a judgment is made on the SIPS summary page as to whether any of these disorders could better account for the clinical picture otherwise being considered to be risk(+).

Final Scoring

Once all the questions have been asked, the patient can join family, spouse, or friends in the waiting room while the interviewer completes the tally of the entire SIPS instrument.

At this point the interviewer uses the information gathered to complete the Global Assessment of Functioning (GAF, pages 229–231), the

Schizotypal Personality Disorder Checklist (page 232), the Summary of SIPS Data (pages 233, 234), and the Summary of SIPS Syndrome Criteria (pages 235, 236).

According to the *Diagnostic and Statistical Manual of Mental Disorders, Fourth Edition* (*DSM–IV*), **Schizotypal Personality Disorder** is a pervasive pattern of social and interpersonal deficits marked by acute discomfort with, and reduced capacity for close relationships as well as by cognitive or perceptual distortions and eccentricities of behavior. Onset can be traced back at least to adolescence or early adulthood. Symptoms are usually "longstanding and stable" although *DSM-IV* does not specify further what this means in terms of months or years. For the SIPS evaluation we have interpreted it to mean one year of stable positive symptoms scoring in the risk syndrome range. This means that new onset positive symptoms in the risk syndrome range are considered at risk, but if they remain stable for one year the diagnosis is changed from risk syndrome to schizotypal. A change in diagnosis can happen in the other direction as well. Someone fulfilling criteria for Schizotypal Personality Disorder may be considered at risk if his "longstanding and stable" symptoms suddenly become worse.

When scoring the GAF section of the SIPS, consider psychological, social, and occupational functioning on a hypothetical continuum of mental health/illness. Do not include impairment in functioning due to physical health or environmental limitations. The interviewer should start at the end of the scale and use it as a checklist to capture the most serious loss of functioning. The checklist is completed twice, once for current state and once for highest level achieved in past year. This will be important when determining the Genetic Risk and Deterioration syndrome.

The SIPS interview is now complete. The scores should be transferred to the last two pages of the SIPS. This is where the diagnostic determination is made. The ratings in each section, the SOPS total score, the personality checklist, and the GAF provide a representation of the patient's overall clinical state. Feedback can now be given to the patient and family, and recommendations for treatment should be based on all of this information.

Chapter 10

Initial Evaluation: Informing Patients and Families of Risk Status and Options

Currently, most help-seeking risk syndrome patients eventually find their way to study centers rather than to specialized treatment clinics. As such, their understanding that their presenting symptoms are also risk markers for psychosis comes from the process of informed consent, a process that focuses initially on the informed consent document. Excerpts of such a document used in the olanzapine clinical trial at the PRIME Clinic in New Haven, Connecticut, are reproduced in Appendix C (pages 237, 238) for illustrative purposes, highlighting the issues of what psychosis is and the risks and benefits of participation in the research.

The risk for psychosis is real, and at the New Haven PRIME Clinic it is conveyed as such. Psychosis is described in terms that are understandable. Its seriousness is acknowledged but counterbalanced with information about the range of potential outcomes including nonpsychotic problems and disorders, the availability of effective treatments, and the fact that these treatments are applied as soon as possible in the event of conversion. The manner in which the clinic deals with knowledge about risk has been discussed in an earlier *Schizophrenia Bulletin* communication and that discussion is reproduced here.[68]

> Our "prodromal" evaluations ascertain both current symptoms and risk for more severe future symptoms (psychosis). Whether the patient is a true risk or a false positive risk, the information we provide may be daunting and unwelcome. The concern

is that imparting such information harbors its own risks, such as generating anxiety, depression, demoralization, panic, or self-stigmatizing behaviors such as withdrawal and isolation.

In actuality, experience in our risk syndrome clinic has been instructive. After we evaluate patients, we tell them (and their family, if appropriate) what we think the problem is, if anything. If they have a problem that does not appear to involve risk, they are so informed, and, if appropriate, a referral is made elsewhere for further evaluation or treatment. If we feel risk is present, we say so and explain why, emphasizing that by "risk" we mean probability, not inevitability. We clarify what we mean by "psychosis," adding that we will have a better picture of the patient's true risk for psychosis, which is why we schedule frequent visits over time. We inform them that should they truly be at risk, they will receive treatment if and when they develop clear signs of psychosis. We add that by being in the study they would probably receive such treatment earlier than if they were being followed in the community. Should they not be at risk for psychosis and develop another disorder instead, we tell them they will receive diagnosis-appropriate referral and treatment right away. We say that if nothing more severe develops over time, the estimate of risk can be revised, bringing to us a better understanding of the source of their original "prodromal" symptoms.

The reactions of patients and their families to this information have ranged from relief to concern to skepticism to denial, the modal response being mixtures of all of these. Distress may be apparent and is usually appropriate to the magnitude of the message. When distress is absent, denial is usually present (but seldom total). To date we have not observed distress that is overwhelming or that requires treatment interventions beyond further information.

We feel that imparting the reality of risks is imparting information that the person may wish to know and may decide is important. When we do this, some patients (and families) also want to know what to do; in our subsequent discussions, they often secure a sense of readiness, perspective, and control by tracking these emerging changes that otherwise are ineffable, puzzling, and potentially disorganizing. Other patients may not achieve such levels of insight and coping. Instead, they deny the reality or level of risk and refuse or withdraw informed consent, or they decide to ignore the reality of risk for the time being but play it safe and join the study. We have seen some form of coping strategy emerge in every case confronted with the news of risk.

Another important concern is that labeling someone as being at risk is stigmatizing, with the label of psychosis becoming a persecutor or a self-fulfilling prophecy. This has not been our experience during our many years of working with this population. In fact, we feel that to avoid imparting the reality of risk is to court even greater stigma from the negative social consequences of active, out-of-control psychotic behavior requiring hospitalization, which is the single most stigmatizing event in the process of onset. Withholding information about risk iatrogenically sanctions denial and places the true positive risk syndrome patient in jeopardy of a potentially disastrous outcome. In our opinion it also violates the patient's civil liberties and right to know.

The anxiety generated by the news of risk can also be a benefit insofar as it heightens vigilance. One feature of this research is the close monitoring of a patient's clinical state, an activity that is maximized if everyone becomes more watchful and knows what to watch for. Greater awareness can also help to identify an emerging psychosis at the time of onset so that treatment is initiated without any delay. Psychosis often arrives like Carl Sandburg's fog; that is, silently, on little cat feet. Its progressive losses and changes are easy to ignore, to explain away, to minimize. Appropriate attention and concern for what is transpiring too often is delayed until the situation spirals into a crisis requiring coercive intervention. First psychosis is a major life crisis; anticipatory anxiety helps to attenuate the shock surrounding onset and its enormous potential for destructive chaos.

What Benefits of Monitoring Are Noted for Psychosis Risk Patients?

Prodromal research, whether or not it includes treatment, has several benefits, both real and potential. First, monitoring and counseling occur on a regular basis, providing continuous feedback about the proband's state of health to patient and family. Troubles, if and when they occur, are apparent right away, and if psychosis supervenes, treatment begins at onset, i.e., at a duration of untreated psychosis of zero. This minimizes the collateral damage and stigma too often generated by untreated irrational behaviors that alienate family, social networks, work colleagues, and sometimes the law. Among the New Haven clinical trial sample of risk syndrome patients who converted to schizophrenia, no patient required hospitalization, all but one continued their daily schedule at work or school, medicine compliance by pill count was 93%, and relationships with family and social networks were maintained.

Research participation offers the opportunity for the patient and family to develop a therapeutic alliance and working relationship with the study clinicians. Engagement with the research and treatment system when competency and decisional capacity are rarely at issue generates trust that is not eroded early or rapidly by emerging psychosis. Another real benefit is the availability of consultation and sometimes treatment for problems comorbid with risk states such as depression, anxiety, or substance abuse. In addition, engagement in risk syndrome research allows for the possibility that preonset tracking and/or treatment will delay or prevent onset or result in a disorder that is milder and less disabling. Finally, a potential benefit important to many risk syndrome participants is the satisfaction that they are adding to the scientific knowledge base about early psychosis.

Chapter 11

Rating Positive and Other Psychosis-Risk Symptoms with the SOPS

The five positive symptoms on which our psychosis-risk assessment rests are Unusual Thought Content (UTC), Suspiciousness/Persecutory Ideas, Grandiose Ideas, Perceptual Abnormalities/Hallucinations, and Disorganized Communication. These can be found on pages 190 to 207 of the SIPS in Appendix B. Each positive symptom has its own section. Each section starts with structured interview questions for probing specific symptomatic experiences characteristic of the symptom. For UTC, characteristic experiences include perplexity and delusional mood, first rank symptoms, overvalued beliefs, other delusions, and non-persecutory ideas of reference. Each characteristic experience is followed by a set of questions to ask the patient. These questions provide clear illustrations in plain language of what is meant by the symptom. For example, first rank symptoms (page 191) are concerned with the origin and ownership of one's thoughts.

Each question is asked during the interview and the patient's response recorded by circling N, NI, or Y. For Yes responses further information is gathered about the symptom to document: when it began, how long it has been active, how frequently it is experienced, and the degree to which the symptom is distressing, disabling, and/or experienced as real.

At the end of the probing question section, the symptom and its component parts are described in detail to help the rater hold in mind the phenomenologies that must be rated on the scale immediately below. The scale, as described earlier, ranges from 0 (absent) to 6 (severe and psychotic). The psychosis-risk range includes scores 3, 4, and 5, and a score of 6 indicates the presence of psychosis.

Each level on the scale contains a descriptive snippet of what a prototypically mild versus moderate versus moderately severe versus severe form of the symptom in question might look like. At the top of the scale the severity of the symptom is anchored by these adjectives, which can be used to rate symptoms that are not easily matched with any of the more detailed level snippets below.

Once a rating is made, the reasons for the rating are documented immediately below the scale. If a symptom is rated in the risk range of severity (level 3–5), then the date of its onset is recorded in the box on the bottom left of the scale page, and if the symptom has gotten worse (by at least one scale point) since onset, the date of that worsening is recorded in the box on the bottom right of the scale page.

For a particular positive symptom to be in the risk range, it must also have *begun* within the past year or, if it began earlier than the past year, then it must have become worse in the past year (i.e., more severe by at least one scale point such as going from a 3 to a 4). This is the reason for recording the date of onset at which the positive symptom reaches a risk level of severity (i.e., at least a 3) or the date at which a pre-existing risk-level symptom becomes worse (by at least one scale point, i.e., it goes from a 3 to a 4 or from a 4 to a 5). Finally, for a particular positive symptom scoring in the 3–5 severity range to actually be a risk symptom, it must happen frequently, specifically an average of at least once a week over the past month.

At this point we will illustrate how these scales can be applied to real (but disguised) case examples of positive symptoms, the aim being to illustrate both the psychopathology characteristic of the psychosis-risk syndrome and the way in which it is measured with the SOPS positive rating scales.

Table 11.1 details actual examples of the five characteristic positive symptoms presented by patients at Yale's psychosis-risk clinic. To the right of each symptom is a brief summary of the SOPS assessment of the vignette, the symptom's rating on the severity scale, and whether or not the symptom is diagnosable as representing risk. Names and identifying characteristics of the patients have been changed to protect anonymity, but the psychopathologic data remain accurate.

Table 11.2 details examples from each of the three "other" SOPS symptom domains: Negative, Disorganization, and General.

Table 11.1 Rater Training Positive Symptom Examples

Positive Symptom 1: Unusual Thought Content	
Case	Interpretation
Elijah stated that he has certain superstitious routines that he must follow before every basketball game to ensure that his team will win the game. For example, he must wear a certain pair of sneakers, put the left one on first, then the right one, then tie the left one and then the right one. He said this began at the beginning of this season and occurs at every game.	• Superstitious beyond what might be expected by average person • Occurs within subculture of athletes • Began within past year (meets criteria that it has begun or worsened in past year) • Occurs at least once a week (meets criteria that it averages once a week over past month) • SOPS rating of this P1=2 • Diagnosable = No (not risk-positive or psychotic)
Dexter (from chapter 9) stated that he spends an increasing amount of time thinking about different ideas and is becoming preoccupied with these ideas. He says that the time he spends thinking about his ideas has increased to more than half the day over the last seven months. He feels that it is important to write these ideas down and to encode them in a private codebook. He carried the codebook with him, showed it to the interviewer and translated the title to the interviewer as "The Book of Ideas." It was written in hieroglyphic-like symbols that the patient said he invented.	• Preoccupation with unusually valued ideas • Not easily dismissed • Has worsened in past year (meets criteria that it has begun or worsened in past year) • Occurs daily (meets criteria that it averages once a week over past month) • P1=3 • Diagnosable = Yes (risk-positive)
Francine's mother described the patient as "more rigid in her thinking about things that don't make sense." Her mother stated that this has intensified over the past two months and occurs at least once a week. She gave the example of Francine describing to her mother a dream in which she was raped. Francine stated that her stomach hurt and she was worried that she might be pregnant. The mother explained that it is not possible to become pregnant from a dream but Francine had a hard time accepting that explanation. Francine acknowledged this experience in the interview and agreed it had been difficult for her to let go of the feeling that she was pregnant. She stated that she knew it wasn't possible but the feeling would not go away and had persisted for at least two weeks. She had trouble concentrating at school because of this dream.	• Thinks ideas or beliefs may be real • Idea that experience may be coming from outside self • Has worsened in the past year (meets criteria that it has begun or worsened in past year) • Occurs at least once a week for several weeks (meets criteria that it averages once a week over past month) • Maintains self-induced skepticism and reality testing • Concentration affected • P1=4 • Diagnosable = Yes (risk-positive)

Continued

Table 11.1 (continued)

Positive Symptom 1: Unusual Thought Content	
Case	Interpretation
Georgia reported that she received special musical radio messages starting three months ago. She often thinks the male artist has written the song specifically about her, like he looked into her head at how she felt and then wrote the song. When questioned if she thought it could be her imagination, she allowed for this possibility but said the feeling can get really strong and sometimes she believes it. This experience occurs daily.	• Belief in reality of mind tricks and mentally triggered events • Belief is compelling and captures attention • Doubt can be induced by others • Has begun in the past year (meets criteria that it has begun or worsened in past year) • Occurs daily for past three months (meets criteria that it averages once a week over past month) • P1=5 • Diagnosable = Yes (risk-positive)
Henry reported that beginning two months ago he sometimes feels as though his classmates can read his mind. He stated that this occurs several times a week in school. He stated that he would have the answer to the teacher's question in his head and then someone else would say the answer. His explanation for this is that he thinks they are reading his mind. He said it feels real to him but he did agree with the interviewer when she suggested that his classmates simply know the answer to the question as well and were not reading his mind. He has recently started avoiding his classmates.	• Compelling belief in reality of mind tricks and magical thinking • Doubt can be induced by another's opinion • Began within last year • Occurs several times a week • Affects social relations • P1=5 • Diagnosable = Yes (risk-positive)
Isaac described an experience that occurred to him a few days prior to the interview and that he has had about five times a week for the past six weeks. He was watching a television program and believed that the characters on the show were somehow in the room with him and interacting with him. He reported that he fully believed in the reality of the experience and that it lasted for the full hour that the show was on TV. When asked how he accounted for the experience, he said he didn't know how they got there but even now he knew that they were all in the room together and interacting with one another. He refused to consider the idea that it might just have been his imagination.	• Unusual thought content with delusional conviction • Attenuation of reality testing even in the context of another's skepticism • Occurs over a period of one month for at least one hour per day at a minimum average frequency of four days per week • P1=6 • Diagnosable = No (psychotic)

Table 11.1 (continued)

Positive Symptom 2: Suspiciousness/Persecutory Ideas	
Case	Interpretation
Jordan stated that occasionally when she walks through the halls at school she feels as though she has to be cautious so that nothing bad happens to her. She could not identify a person, persons, or thing that she thought might harm her, just a vague sense of feeling unsafe. This feeling began eight months ago.	• Occasional doubts about safety • Hyper-vigilance without a clear source of danger • Started within past year • P2=2 • Diagnosable = No
Karl stated that at least twice a week, beginning six months ago, he has the feeling that other people are thinking about him in a negative manner. He stated that he can tell by the way they stare at him and then quickly turn away. He also reported a vague feeling that he is being watched. These feelings occur about twice a week but he stated that he knows they are not real.	• Recurrent sense that people are thinking negatively about him • Unfounded or exaggerated • Began within past year • Occurs occasionally • Uncomfortable for him even if not real • P2=3 • Diagnosable = Yes (risk-positive)
Lyle reported that several times a week in the past four months he has had recurrent feelings that people are talking about him and occasional fears that some people may want to harm him. He reported that he typically tells himself to "disregard it," but his suspiciousness remains and he feels unsafe much of the time. He reported confronting a few people at work about this to see if it was an accurate perception but they denied that they were talking about him	• Clear thoughts of being singled out • Sense that people intend to harm him • Self-induced doubt through reality checks • Occurs regularly • Began in past year • P2=4 • Diagnosable = Yes (risk-positive)
Mike reported that he thinks people think negatively about him and are plotting to make him confess everything that he has ever done wrong. He also thinks that people at work make fun of him for not knowing as much as they do. Recently he became agitated at work because he suspected some of his coworkers might be undercover cops. His supervisor noticed how anxious he was and sent him home for the rest of the day. When questioned whether he really believed they were cops, he stated that he knew it wasn't true but it felt so real that he became confused. This began several months ago and occurs several times a week.	• Concern about plots • Behavior affected • Occurs several times a week • Began within past year • Reality tests with help • P2=5 • Diagnosable = Yes (risk-positive)

Continued

Table 11.1 (continued)

Positive Symptom 2: Suspiciousness/Persecutory Ideas	
Case	Interpretation
Nathaniel reported that he thinks his friend hacked into his computer six months ago and stole his password and his identity. He also thinks that his friend used a web cam to take pictures of him jumping nude into a lake and that he and other friends are circulating these pictures on Facebook. He stated that he thinks it started as a prank but now is vicious and malicious. He stated that he felt betrayed by his friends even though they deny these things. He said that he is absolutely confident the hacking has occurred and that people are spreading the picture and messages about him. This happens every time he goes on his computer. He now avoids these friends and spends more time alone at home.	• Convinced about plots, no doubt • Persistent and pervasive • Affects social behavior • Began within past year • P2=6 • Diagnosable = No (psychotic)

Positive Symptom 3: Grandiosity	
Case	Interpretation
Opal stated that she has special talents but she is not sure what they are. She stated that she plans to be a playwright and has written one play and is working on two others. Two months ago she saw an ad on E-Bay for a used bus and wanted to bid on it so she could travel the country and perform her play. She said it was an impulsive thought and she did not continue pursuing it.	• Thoughts, fantasies of success • Kept to self • Not lasting or persistent • P3=2 • Diagnosable = No (not risk-positive or psychotic)
Prescott is a 13-year-old eighth grader. He stated, "I don't mean to brag but I tend to think in a wide way, with variety and color, like in a worldly, mature way." He reported that he has "excellent strategy" at computer games. He says he has the reading level of an 18-year-old and that he is planning to write a Tolkien-type book. He stated that he started feeling this way nine months ago and it occurs nearly everyday.	• Expansive • Notions of being unusually gifted or special • Occurs at least once a week over past month • Began or worsened in past year • P3=3 • Diagnosable = Yes (risk-positive)

Table 11.1 (continued)

Positive Symptom 3: Grandiosity	
Case	Interpretation
Quenton reported the belief that he possesses special talents with his *Yu-Gi-Oh!* Cards. He said that he started being good at it around this past Christmas and that he is getting better and better every day. He stated he is very good at receiving special messages from the cards about other people in his life. When asked whether anyone else could receive these messages, he stated that no one else has these special talents and therefore no one else can receive messages from the cards. However, he said that it may be possible for someone else to develop the same level of skill that he possesses if they were to spend a great deal of time studying the cards.	• Loosely organized beliefs of special talents or abilities • Spontaneously offered that other people might be able to do the same if they practiced • Began within past year • Occurs at least once a week in past month • P3=4 • Diagnosable = Yes (risk-positive)
Reardon reported that he runs very fast to the extent that he can keep up with a car, that he can make fire move just by looking at it, and that he has enough power in his punches to dent a metal door. He said he is not 100 percent convinced of these things and that if someone measured his speed and said it was normal or if someone said it was just the fire flickering or said that others could dent the door as well, he would easily believe it. These beliefs began about four months ago.	• Several special talents • Unreal and unusual • Frequent • Skepticism can be induced by others • P3=5 • Diagnosable = Yes (risk-positive)
Sarah reported that she has the power to heal. For example, if she gets a cut she can focus on it and it will heal extra fast. She stated that she can't heal others but only herself. She stated that she believes it 100 percent and she doesn't worry about injuries because she knows that she can heal herself. She suspected she had this power about six months ago but now knows for certain that it is true.	• Power to heal • Delusional conviction • P3=6 • Diagnosable = No (psychotic)

Continued

Table 11.1 (continued)

Positive Symptom 4: Perceptual Abnormalities	
Case	Interpretation
Therese reported that about once a month she hears noise in her head that sounds like voices. They are vague and she cannot distinguish what they are saying, if anything. This usually happens when she is very stressed or tired.	• Noise inside head • Unclear • Stress and fatigue related • P4=2 • Diagnosable = No
Ursula stated that she hears her name being called about three times per month. This experience has begun in the past year and she is uncertain what to make of it. She reported that when she hears her name being called she often turns to look or asks someone if they heard it too.	• Persistent auditory perceptual distortion • Experienced as unusual and somewhat worrisome so that she does a reality check • Began within past year • Occurs three times a month • P4=3 • Diagnosable = No (it does not meet the average frequency requirement of once a week)
Vince reported that at times he thinks he hears something in the next room, like people inside the garage or the garage door opening or someone calling his name. He stated that he goes to look and there is no one there. He reported that these experiences currently occur about once a week. He also reported visual illusions such as seeing a door opening slightly, something running across the floor, or the silhouette of a person standing nearby. These experiences happen about three times a week and began four months ago. He attributed these experiences to "lighting or shadows."	• Recurrent formed illusions or momentary hallucinations • Recognized as not being real • Somewhat captivating • Began within last year • Occurs at least once a week • P4=4 • Diagnosable = Yes (risk-positive)
Walton reported that every time he goes into his art class, twice a week, the pictures of leopards and birds on the walls suddenly become "3D—like they are moving." He stated that the pictures first appear to move around in the frames, then leave the frames and fly around the room. He stated that he sees them in a shadowy way, not the way he sees other things. This experience began at the beginning of the school year. When questioned, he reported that he knows it is not real although it feels very real to him. He is not sure of the source of the experience.	• Recurrent momentary hallucinations • Recognized as not real yet captivating • Not sure of source of experience • Began within last year • Occurs at least once a week • P4=5 • Diagnosable = Yes (risk-positive)

Table 11.1 (continued)

Positive Symptom 4: Perceptual Abnormalities	
Case	Interpretation
Xavier reported that several times a week, wherever he may be, he hears a voice call his name and start talking to him. He hears the voice clearly just like he hears the interviewer's voice. He said it makes him angry when he looks around and doesn't see anyone. The voice taunts him so that he can't attend to what he is doing, and he has no control over it. This started four months ago and happens almost daily. It interferes with his ability to concentrate. He knows the voice is real even though he can't see the person.	• Persistent, clear, external voice • No doubt • Almost daily • Affects concentration • Diagnosable = No (psychotic)

Positive Symptom 5: Disorganized Communication	
Case	Interpretation
Yvette reported occasional communication difficulties such as making a comment that doesn't fit during conversations with her friends. During our interview she asked that I repeat a few questions because she was unclear of the meaning but her speech was organized and she was easy to understand.	• Occasional irrelevancies by report • Not seen in interview • P5=2 • Diagnosable = No
Zenia stated that people sometimes tell her they cannot understand her when she speaks. She reported that she talks in circles. During the interview she rambled occasionally and required some redirection from the interviewer. She reports that this happens every day and it has occurred ever since she began talking and is not getting worse.	• Going off track • Occasional irrelevant topics • Responds to clarifying questions • Longstanding and stable • P5=3 • Diagnosable = No (because symptom is not new)
Antoine reports that his friends have a great deal of difficulty following him when he tries to explain things to them. During the interview he had difficulty getting to the point but eventually he did. Through direct and structured questioning he was able to answer the questions correctly. Antoine stated that this began after Thanksgiving, happens on a daily basis, and is very frustrating to him.	• Circumstantial speech • Difficulty directing answers toward the goal • Redirectable through structured questioning • Began within last year • Occurs daily • P5=4 • Diagnosable = Yes (risk-positive)

Continued

Table 11.1 (continued)

Positive Symptom 5: Disorganized Communication	
Case	**Interpretation**
Biff's communication was very slow during the interview, and he had significant difficulty directing his sentences to the point. The patient was aware of his difficulty communicating and said that he mentally reviews what he plans to say a couple of times before speaking but often forgets anyway. Several times during the interview he would trail off onto another topic and when asked about this said that he forgot the question. He appeared distressed when this happened. He could be redirected briefly with structured questions.	• Tangential loss of focus • Aware of/distressed by problems communicating • Organization needs repeated prompts • P5=5 • Diagnosable = Yes
Claire was not responsive to the structured questions during the interview. She spoke on irrelevant topics throughout the interview and the topics themselves were not related. Occasional loose associations. She could not be redirected with prompts and did not follow even very simple questions.	• Loose associations • Not redirectable with questions • P5=6 • Diagnosable = No (psychotic)

Table 11.2 Rater Training "Other" Symptom Examples

Negative Symptom 1: Social Anhedonia	
Case	**Interpretation**
Therese (this chapter) said she prefers to be alone and is uncomfortable with groups of people. She waits for others to contact her but once there does enjoy socializing.	• Interpersonally passive • Resistant to engagement • Responsive once involved • N1=2
Corine (Chapter 7) reports that she rarely sees people outside of work. In fact, she has noticed that people have stopped asking her to join them and she doesn't even miss it. This is a change because prior to several months ago, she had three or four friends from work and she saw them in social settings several times a week.	• Few friends • Social apathy • Minimal social participation because of disinterest, not because of shyness or social anxiety • N1=4
Damian reported that he is a loner and does not have any friends. He stated that he never does things with friends outside of school and doesn't really socialize even in school. He stated that he would not be more social even given the opportunity.	• Hermetic • No friends in any context • Prefers isolation • N1=6

Table 11.2 (continued)

Negative Symptom 2: Avolition	
Case	Interpretation
Eunice and her parents noted that she is uncharacteristically having more difficulty finishing tasks and following through with directions. She says that she's having problems getting motivated.	• Lagging effort • New, perhaps temporary • N2=1
Prescott (Chapter 11) reports that nearly every day since the start of this school year he has had difficulty getting himself motivated to do things. He has energy but less interest in getting normal activities done. He says that he manages but that his mom or his teacher often have to prod him to initiate or finish a task.	• Low level of motivation, not low level of energy • Difficulty starting tasks • Difficulty finishing tasks • Requires occasional prodding • N2=3
Fred reports that he has difficulty getting motivated to do things that he does not see the point to do, which is almost everything except his computer games. Prodding from friends and family usually falls flat.	• No interest in productive endeavors • Nonresponsive to the wishes/demands of others • N2=6
Negative Symptom 3: Expression of Emotion	
Case	Interpretation
Gabby seemed quiet and distant until the tear down her cheek became apparent.	• Affectively alive • Shy or modest • N3=1
Harold answered questions and asked a few himself, but both answers and questions were brief and stilted. He seemed bored.	• Engaged formally • Feeling of distance • N3=3
Inez appeared very flat during the interview. She responded with one-word answers when the interviewer asked leading questions. She did not smile or laugh, frown or cry, or use any hand gestures during the entire interview.	• Constricted affect • Flat, minimally responsive • Lack of gestures, expression • N3=5
Negative Symptom 4: Experience of Emotion and Self	
Case	Interpretation
Julianna complained that she has not been able to get excited about her friends and boyfriend recently. She says it's like coming down with a fever and wanting to stay in bed.	• Reduced enthusiasm • Unwelcome change • Probably temporary • N4=1

Continued

Table 11.2 (continued)

Negative Symptom 4: Experience of Emotion and Self	
Case	Interpretation
Keth reported that he was not his usual self, as if part of him was missing. He reported feeling disconnected from everything but found people's concern for him strange. He stated he felt emotionally flat and often could not tell what he was feeling.	• Missing self • Not connected internally and externally • Flat or undifferentiated affect • N4=5

Negative Symptom 5: Ideational Richness	
Case	Interpretation
Louisa reported that she occasionally found it hard to follow conversations because she felt people had their own way of saying something that others understood but that she didn't.	• Not "with it" or comfortably present and fluid with the prevailing conversation and/or topic • N5=2
It was noted that Henry (Chapter 11) had difficulty following even uncomplicated parts of the interview. He missed two of the similarities and did provide some concrete interpretations for the proverbs.	• Concrete interpretation of proverbs • Misses nuances in conversations • Doesn't get the "gist" • N5=4
Marcus was unable to keep up with the interview. He nodded yes or no answers but could not provide any additional information or opinions. He looked like he did not understand what was being talked about. The interviewer made multiple attempts to gather the information but with no results.	• Present physically but not mentally or emotionally • N5=6

Negative Symptom 6: Occupational Functioning	
Case	Interpretation
Noah reports that he is still earning high honors in school, getting grades in the A and B range. However, in the last three months he has noticed that he is having more and more trouble with his work. He stated that the work is not harder, it is just that it takes him more effort to get it done.	• Maintaining usual level of functioning • Taking more effort than usual • Change occurring in last few months • N6=1
Ozzie reported a drop in his grade point average. He stated that his work takes more time than it use to, like with his home chores each day. He is experiencing difficulty getting things done.	• Drop in work capacity, productivity • Change reflected in grades or job performance, i.e., noticeable • N6=3

Table 11.2 (continued)

Negative Symptom 6: Occupational Functioning	
Case	**Interpretation**
Paige reported three suspensions from school this marking period. She is having uncharacteristic difficulty making up her work and is at risk of failing some classes. She knows this is happening but does not seem to know how to turn things around.	• Failure in several areas • Struggles seem new and unusual for her • N6=5
Disorganization Symptom 1: Odd Behavior or Appearance	
Case	**Interpretation**
Qevia came to the interview in a 50s skirt. She said she borrowed it from her mother. She was nervous and wanted to present herself as a young lady.	• Slightly off-setting appearance • Unusual quality recognized and an explanation given • D1=2
Roger presented in an all black punk wardrobe and mumbled to himself on more than one occasion about being a priest of dark rituals and alchemy.	• Unusual presentation and demeanor • Counterculture, quasi-religious ideation • D1=4
Samantha presented at the interview in a lovely spring dress, wearing a straw hat that was completely lined with aluminum foil. She had plastic wrap around her hands and her shoes and large wads of cotton protruding from her ears.	• Grossly strange appearance • Unusual in ways outside the norm or culture • D1=6
Disorganization Symptom 2: Bizarre Thinking	
Case	**Interpretation**
Henry (Chapter 11) thought that telepathy could have powerful effects on the weather and seismic activity in unstable ecosystems, like Yellowstone Park. He gave extended descriptions of how it worked if asked.	• Persistent, unusual thinking • Unconventional, idiosyncratic beliefs • D2=4
Travis reported in the interview that during the previous night while he watched Jay Leno on TV, a force switched his brain with Leno's and now he could only think like Leno and not like himself.	• Ideas that are patently absurd and violate the laws of nature • D2=6

Continued

Table 11.2 (continued)

Disorganization Symptom 3: Trouble with Focus and Attention	
Case	Interpretation
Ule reports that he gets distracted easily. He states that sometimes his daydreaming interferes with his ability to focus on tasks and conversations. He said that this has been happening persistently since the start of the school year.	• Distracted frequently • Inattention caused by daydreaming • On and off since start of school year • D3=3
Valerie had difficulty responding to the questions throughout the interview. She would lose track of the conversation and needed direct questions to regain her focus.	• Loses track of conversation • Requires others to refocus • D3=5

Disorganization Symptom 4: Impairment in Personal Hygiene	
Case	Interpretation
Wanda reports that she is not as interested in her clothes or her appearance as in the past. It is not as important to her that she wear makeup and fix her hair, but she still showers everyday.	• Not as interested in physical appearance • Less concerned with social conventions about makeup and hair • Maintains personal hygiene • D4=2
Xander appeared somewhat unkempt and reported that he only showers once a week. There was no apparent odor present.	• Persistent but not total neglect of hygiene • D4=4
Yogi appeared disheveled and dirty. His clothes were stained and there was a distinct odor about him. His hair was unwashed and uncombed. When his self-care was questioned he shrugged and changed the subject.	• Total neglect of body and wardrobe • Unresponsive to intervention • D4=6

General Symptom 2: Dysphoric Mood	
Case	Interpretation
Zachary reports that he has not been feeling like himself lately. He reports that he has been feeling sad for no apparent reason. He cries easily and has been feeling anxious. Such feelings are new to him but he says it is like "the blues have come to stay."	• Feeling sad, blue, anxious • First time, but not going away • G2=3
Annabelle reported feeling sad and bad, anxious and irritable for most of the time. She reported difficulty coping with these feelings and spends a great deal of time sleeping to avoid these feelings.	• Mixed negative affects • Tries to escape in sleep • G2=5

Table 11.2 (continued)

General Symptom 4: Impaired Tolerance to Natural Stress	
Case	Interpretation
Brayden stated he does not worry a great deal but does find himself tired at the end of his day even if nothing unusual occurred.	• More tired than usual • No cause for concern • G4=1
Carlos reports that he gets thrown off by unexpected things that happen to him during the day. He reports feeling overwhelmed by his school work, he gets anxious, and experiences catastrophic thinking. He reports that this has been occurring on a daily basis since the beginning of the school year.	• Is overwhelmed on a daily basis by stressful situations that he used to handle as a matter of course • Is anxious but does not have panic attacks • Began within past year • G4=5

Chapter 12

Rating Actual Cases, Baseline Assessment

This chapter provides descriptions of thirteen cases coming to psychosis-risk clinics for their baseline assessment. They have gone through the screening process and the SIPS, SCID, or KSADS[69], and an Axis II interview, and have provided enough history, behaviors, and symptoms to render a judgment as to whether they meet criteria for the risk syndrome, for psychosis, or are help-seeking controls who may be struggling with one or more other psychiatric disorders.

The case illustrations or "write-ups" contain a great deal of condensed information and are presented here as they are presented to the research teams in our risk syndrome clinics. These cases are real but carefully disguised. Key demographic information (age, gender, ethnicity) have been altered to mask personal identity.

The cases have been selected and will be presented by their SIPS diagnostic status for pedagogical reasons. Here we are interested, for example, in illustrating what a moderate risk case looks like at initial (baseline) evaluation and how it differs from a mild and/or a moderately severe case, or how it differs from a patient already psychotic.

Once again, these are real cases as they presented at baseline. Chapter 14 will illustrate some of the typical ways psychosis-risk patients progress over time. Chapter 15 will present another large number of baseline evaluations, this time without their SOPS scores. You will provide the scores, and then compare them with those given to the patient by the evaluation team. The latter are at the end of Chapter 15, which you are encouraged not to visit until your own evaluations are complete.

The case write-ups follow (sometimes loosely) the following protocol: patient demographics, chief complaint, referral source, past medical and psychiatric treatment history, family history (especially of psychiatric disorders), substance use/abuse history, significant birth/developmental history, functional and cognitive capacities over time up to the evaluation, and the presence of other Axis I or Axis II psychiatric disorders as obtained by administering other structured diagnostic interviews. Finally, given that the SOPS positive symptom scores are central to the risk diagnosis, the scores of these key ratings and the reasons for each rating are provided. Scores of other symptom sets (negative, disorganization, general) are elaborated for illustrative purposes, especially if noteworthy, but the primary focus is on the positive symptoms, which are required for the diagnostic determination. Also of particular interest is whether there has been a significant change in functional capacity in the recent past. This is usually captured by major differences in the Global Assessment of Functioning scale over the past year.

All of this information is routinely gathered during the typical baseline risk evaluation and all of it is presented at the diagnostic conference. Not all of it will be reproduced in our cases here, however. In the interest of parsimony and pedagogy only the discriminating diagnostic clinical data will be presented. Therefore, a lack of information, e.g., concerning grandiosity for example, does not mean it was ignored. It means it was asked about and found not to be diagnostically pivotal.

This chapter will present illustrative cases for the following diagnostic categories: Attenuated Positive Symptom (APS) Psychosis-Risk Syndrome: levels 3, 4, and 5, post-psychotic syndrome (Residual); Brief Intermittent Psychotic State (BIPS); Genetic Risk and Deterioration State (GRD); Schizotypal Personality Disorder (STPD), and Help-Seeking Controls (HSC) or persons who are symptomatic and treatment seeking but who do not meet the criteria for any risk(+) syndrome. They are called "controls" because such people are often recruited into follow-along studies of risk(+) populations as non-risk(+) comparison or "control" cases.

Case 1
Subject ID: Dominica

BACKGROUND AND PRESENTING INFORMATION: Dominica is a 16-year-old Hispanic female living in a group home since two months ago. She attends high school, where she is in a program for students who are quite far behind in their studies. She is also looking for part-time work. Throughout her life, she has had a series of unstable housing situations—first with her mother, then her father, then foster care, and then at the age of 10 she returned to live with her mother, who "kicked her out" at 15, so she lived for a short time in her own apartment.

CHIEF COMPLAINT: The staff at the group home referred Dominica because they were concerned about her "confusing" conversational style (jumping from topic to topic), episodes of staring into space, and suicidal ideation.

PAST TREATMENT HISTORY: She receives individual counseling through a youth organization. She was taken to a hospital ER one month ago by the group home staff for expressing suicidal ideation. She was determined to be chronically dysfunctional, of very low risk, and she was discharged.

FAMILY HISTORY: Dominica's mother has been diagnosed with schizophrenia and with significant alcohol and marijuana use. There are no reports of mental illness or substance abuse in any other family members.

CURRENT AND PAST SUBSTANCE USE: Extensive, beginning with marijuana use at the age of 13. She spent much of her 14th and 15th year using some kind of substance—including alcohol, marijuana, amphetamines, mushrooms, ecstasy, and rarely, morphine. She continues to use alcohol and marijuana a few times a week and ecstasy on occasion.

SCID: Past marijuana dependence, starting age 14, early partial remission.

Past hallucinogen dependence, early partial remission.

DIPD: Nil.

Current/Highest GAF in Past Year: 48/50

SOPS RATINGS:

P1. Unusual Thought Content: Dominica has had occasional (once a month for the last two months) vague ideas of reference. For example, she once saw a matchbox from a club she had been to on the ground far from the club and had the thought "What I do does not go unnoticed." She had no clear idea of who might be noticing.

P1=1

P2. Suspiciousness:

Denied suspiciousness and is quite careless with her personal safety even though she feels that people are not very trustworthy. She seemed somewhat guarded in revealing some of her more personal information.

P2=2

P3. Grandiosity:

Dominica described herself as really good "at a lot of things" but could only give "building things" as an example. She told this interviewer that she wanted to be an obstetrician. She was aware that her academic standing would need to improve significantly in order for this to happen.

P3=1

P4. Perceptual Abnormalities/Hallucinations:

She endorses noticing sounds sounding different at certain pitches. She was not able to provide much detail. She notices this every day.

P4=1

P5. Disorganized Communication:

Responses to questions were a little odd at times, as they could be vague or cryptic. She said that occasionally she "blabbers," but this was not observed in the interview.

P5=2

N1. Social Anhedonia:

N1=0

N5. Decreased Ideational Richness:

N5=0

Psychosis-Risk State: Help-Seeking Control (HSC) with past substance use problems and a positive family history for psychosis.

Case 2

Subject ID: Earl

BACKGROUND AND PRESENTING INFORMATION: Earl is a 13-year-old African American male who is in the seventh grade of middle school. He lives with his biological mother and father, and a 15-year-old sister. He was referred to the risk syndrome clinic because of a recent increase in school-peer-related behavioral outbursts, and anxieties and depression associated with those peers.

REFERRAL SOURCE: The patient was referred by a psychiatrist who is familiar with the risk syndrome clinic, and who was concerned about Earl's increase in behavioral problems and their being associated with some unusual thoughts.

PAST PSYCHIATRIC HISTORY: The patient has never been psychiatrically hospitalized. He recently began psychotherapy with a psychologist and he has been seeing a psychiatrist for emotional outbursts starting at age nine. Medicine (Strattera) was prescribed for the first time six months ago.

CURRENT AND PAST SUBSTANCE USE: He reported no alcohol or substance use or experimentation.

SIGNIFICANT DEVELOPMENTAL AND MEDICAL DETAILS: Earl's mother had a normal pregnancy with good prenatal care per her report. She had not used any alcohol or other substances during her pregnancy. Delivery was by scheduled C-section due to a previous C-section delivery. The infant was born in good health and without any physical concerns. Most developmental milestones were reached on time and there were no significant health matters during early childhood.

By age two, however, it was apparent that Earl was not developing speech normatively. He received speech therapy and social group services from age two until age six (first grade). He did not receive a diagnosis for these difficulties, despite workups, and did not attend special education.

No suggestion of an autism-spectrum disorder was made, but the patient and his mother did endorse some of the signs of autism during the baseline assessment, but they were below the threshold for concern and referral. Nevertheless, it was also clear that some of his difficulties with behavioral dyscontrol began in early childhood.

Earl was always quite intelligent and did very well academically in school, although he continued to have difficulty in understanding how his actions or statements affected others. His excellent academic performance was regularly punctuated with interpersonal difficulties. He experienced a significant worsening of these outbursts along with anxiety, depression, and an increase in unusual thoughts starting six months ago.

MEDICATION HISTORY: He began Strattera 40 mg/day for ADHD six months ago.

FAMILY HISTORY OF MENTAL/SUBSTANCE ABUSE DISORDERS: Earl's mother is diagnosed with a depressive disorder. His father is being treated for possible adult ADHD. His sister is diagnosed with dysthymic disorder.

OTHER DIAGNOSES: Earl did meet DSM-IV lifetime criteria for Depressive Disorder NOS in remission, and Attention Deficit Hyperactivity Disorder, current. He did not meet criteria for any personality disorder on the DIPD instrument, including Schizotypal Personality Disorder.

Current/Highest GAF in Past Year: 53/61

SUMMARY OF SOPS RATINGS:

The patient reported a **moderate level of unusual thought content/ delusional ideas**. He daydreams a lot and is sometimes bored. He stated that boring situations last longer since around eight months ago and that fun things happen more slowly since one year ago. He believes that monkeys will likely rule the world someday because they were the first to travel in space and would therefore have been likely to have made an alliance with an alien civilization. This belief began about three years ago, but he thinks about it more and more, especially since eight months ago. He does not have delusional conviction about the monkeys, however, but stated that he thinks about it as being very possible. These experiences and beliefs are only mildly distressing.

P1=3

The patient reported a **mild level of suspiciousness/persecutory ideas**. He said he doesn't necessarily trust that people will do things, such as return a game they might have borrowed. He suspects people would like to steal his "stuff" if given the chance.

P2=2

The patient reported a **questionably present level of grandiosity**. He stated that he is smart in school, good at video games and at time management.

P3=1

The patient reported **a moderate level of perceptual abnormalities**. Some type of auditory experience occurs about one time per week. These began eight months ago but worsened four months ago and are mildly distressing. He sometimes hears the phone or doorbell ring when no one is there. He sometimes hears his name being called when no one has actually called him. He experiences these sounds as being just as real and clear as a voice from an actual person. He will likely look out the window or pick up the phone in response to these experiences.

P4=3

The patient reported a **questionably present level of disorganized communication**. He stated that he sometimes over-elaborates, and this was observed during the interview.

P5=1

The patient reported a **questionably present level of social anhedonia**. He has 10 to 15 friends, enjoys their company, but sees them outside of school only about one time per week and admits that he often likes to be alone.

N1=1

Conclusion: Based on the level 3 ratings for P1 and P4, which began or worsened within the past year and were occurring on an average frequency of once per month, Earl meets criteria as an APS Psychosis-Risk Syndrome.

Case 3

Subject ID: Felicity

DEMOGRAPHICS: Felicity is a 23-year-old, single, mixed racial female college student who transferred last year from a small, two-year college. She found adjusting to a larger school quite stressful and has had a drop in her grades. She is living at home with her parents while attending school, and this is a major source of stress for her. She recently left a long-term relationship that was abusive.

CHIEF COMPLAINT: Felicity responded to an informational e-mail from the local risk syndrome clinic. She had concerns about unusual thoughts she was experiencing recently.

PAST PSYCHIATRIC HISTORY: She reports a history of depression and anxiety beginning in elementary school. She was never hospitalized but had outpatient treatment with multiple trials of antidepressants including Zoloft, Effexor, Wellbutrin, Celexa, and most recently Prozac. She has a history of cutting behaviors beginning in middle school with the last cutting episode being two years ago. She reports a history of childhood sexual abuse.

PAST MEDICAL HISTORY: Unremarkable.

SUBSTANCE ABUSE HISTORY: None

FAMILY PSYCHIATRIC HISTORY: Felicity reports a significant history of depression and anxiety throughout her family including her mother, two sisters, maternal uncles, and maternal grandmother. She reports some paranoia in a sister and maternal grandmother.

SCID: Major Depression, recurrent, Post-Traumatic Stress Disorder, Obsessive-Compulsive Disorder.

DIPD: Borderline Personality Disorder, no Schizotypal Personality Disorder.

Current/Highest GAF in the Past Year: 60/60.

SUMMARY OF SOPS RATINGS.

Moderately Severe Level of Unusual Thought Content: Felicity reports that beginning this year, and happening several times a month, she feels as if her friends are different people than who they are supposed to be. She does not think they are really different, but finds the experience unsettling, as if she has been displaced into a "different reality" where everything seems different and alien.

She reports longstanding déjà vu experiences several times a month, and in about one-third of these occurrences she feels she actually predicts correctly what will happen next. She states this is probably just intuition and finds it annoying but not disturbing. She has a longstanding superstition that if you kill a spider something terrible will happen to you and she will not kill a spider even if it is dangerous. She reports longstanding and daily feelings as if things happening around her have a special meaning. For example, she saw a bird caught in a power line and saw a similar tattoo of a bird on a friend, which she took to mean that she should date this person. She states that everything happens for a reason and that fate gives you universal clues about how things are supposed to be. This influences her behavior to some degree.

Felicity reports a new experience over the past six weeks of thinking that bugs are communicating with her. It now happens at least weekly. She states she doesn't actually hear anything but she has a physical sensation as if she has heard something. She describes that when near an insect she will get the sensation as if she has heard something in her mind like "I'm waiting," or "I am what I am." This usually lasts for seconds to minutes. Last Saturday she had a similar experience with an inanimate object (a deer skull), which she felt told her its name. She finds this bothersome, worrisome, and makes her wonder if she is "going crazy."

P1=4

Mild level of Suspiciousness: Felicity reports being wary about who is around her, where exits are located, etc. These experiences are longstanding and stable. She reports occasionally she might see people laughing and wonder if they are laughing at her. Also longstanding.

P2=2

Absence of Grandiose Ideas.

P3=0

Moderate Level of Perceptual Abnormalities: Felicity reports hearing her name being called and/or what sounds like people talking, "an impression of voices," one time every few months. This has been longstanding and stable. Once a month she feels pressure as if a person is pushing on her back, wonders if it could be a spiritual entity "hitching a ride." She finds this mostly annoying but scary at times. She sees lights or shadows out of the corner of her eye, or movement under the door when no one is there. She does not find this bothersome. It is longstanding but has been increasing to a weekly happening in the past two months.

P4=3

Mild Level of Disorganized Communication: Felicity reports over the past several months that she will sometimes catch herself rambling in conversation. Her communication was not disorganized during the interview, however.

P5=2

N1= 0 No Social Anhedonia

N5=0 No Decreased Ideational Richness:

Summary: Individual meets criteria for an APS Psychosis-Risk Syndrome, based on P1 and P4.

Case 4

Subject ID: Garth

BACKGROUND INFORMATION: Garth is an 18-year-old Caucasian male. He resides with his parents and younger sister. He is currently in the 12th grade in high school. He earns As and Bs, is on the honor roll, and participates in wrestling and the debate team.

REFERRAL SOURCE: The patient was referred to the risk syndrome clinic by a psychiatrist in the area.

PRESENTING ISSUE: The parents report that it was like their son hit a brick wall. One day he was doing fine, on the honor roll, captain of the wrestling team, and socially active with a longstanding girlfriend. The next day he reported hearing a voice two to three times a week that would say negative things to him. The patient reports that the voice is getting louder and meaner and it scares him. In addition, he is beginning to have some "dark," unusual ideas that trouble him. These symptoms are interfering with his ability to function in school and within his social circle.

PAST PSYCHIATRIC HISTORY: The patient has no prior history of emotional difficulties or psychiatric treatment.

CURRENT AND PAST SUBSTANCE USE: The patient did not report any substance experimentation or use or abuse.

SIGNIFICANT MEDICAL HISTORY: The patient reports no significant childhood illnesses other than chicken pox.

MEDICATION HISTORY: The patient has never been prescribed psychiatric medications.

FAMILY HISTORY OF MENTAL/SUBSTANCE ABUSE DISORDERS: The patient and his parents report that his maternal grandfather was diagnosed with chronic Paranoid Schizophrenia and a paternal uncle was also diagnosed with psychosis.

OTHER DIAGNOSES: The patient did not meet SCID criteria for any Axis I disorder. He did not meet criteria on the DIPD for any Axis II disorder.

Current/Highest GAF in Past Year: 55/90

SUMMARY OF SOPS RATINGS:

The patient reported a **severe but not psychotic level of unusual thought content.** He reported that conversations play over and over in his head and he gets confused between which are real and which are imaginary. This is occurring on a daily basis since its onset two months ago. He reports that it interferes with his ability to focus and attend to conversations and to things happening around him. He also stated that it interferes with his relationships because he reacts to people as if these conversations are real. In fact, he stated that he and his girlfriend broke up because of it. He wonders if this is a result of some type of external mind control trying to mess with his life. Upon direct questioning, he could acknowledge that this might just be his mind playing tricks on him.

P1=5

Garth reported **a severe but not psychotic level of suspiciousness**. He reports that he thinks people are talking about him in a negative way. He believes that people are "out to get him" and want to ruin his life and his happiness. He appeared guarded and stated frequently that you must always be watchful because there is danger all around. While the patient did not dismiss these beliefs easily, skepticism could be induced. He reports that this began two months ago and occurs on a daily basis.

P2=5

The patient did not report any signs or symptoms of **grandiosity**.

P3=0

He reported a **severe but not psychotic level of perceptual abnormalities**. Two months ago the patient reported hearing noises that sound like voices. At first this was very subtle, but it has grown in intensity. He states that the voices say mean and nasty things and that he is often frightened by the voices. He is unclear whether the voices are only in his head or if they are outside his head. This occurs at least four to five times a week. He finds this experience confusing and skepticism as to its reality could be induced.

P4=5

The patient did not report or exhibit signs and symptoms of **disorganized communication**.

P5=0

Psychosis-Risk State: Based upon the rating for P1, P2, and P4, Garth meets criteria for an APS Psychosis-Risk Syndrome. All symptoms started two months ago and occur on a weekly basis. Despite a GAF loss of more than 30% in the past year and a history of psychosis in the family, Garth does not meet criteria for the Genetic Risk and Deterioration risk syndrome because there is no diagnosed psychosis in any first-degree relative.

Case 5

Subject ID: Helen

IDENTIFYING DATA: Helen is a 22-year-old single, Asian female, recent college graduate. She self-referred to our psychosis-risk service because of a series of unusual thoughts and experiences which began a number of years ago but which have been increasing over the last 6–12 months. Over the past year she has been in therapy and taking

antidepressants for depression and anxiety, but states that this was not too helpful.

FAMILY PSYCHIATRIC HISTORY: Father—mildly paranoid for years but without decline in function or other psychotic symptoms or treatment. Mother—periods of mild paranoia and visual hallucinations (e.g., trails of light), very moody and irritable, consistent work history, no psychiatric treatment. Sister—age 25 and healthy.

SCID: Generalized Anxiety Disorder.

DIPD: Nil.

Current/Highest GAF in Past Year: 55/65

SIPS/SOPS Ratings

Unusual Thought Content: Onset two years ago but worse four months ago.

Believes with delusional conviction (two occasions for up to 15 minutes each time) that there are aliens that want her to do bad things (break things, vandalize), and cheer her on when she gets angry. Notices coincidences a few times per week. Occasional (monthly) episodes of fearing that her boyfriend is imaginary, e.g., at a movie with him she goes to the restroom and is fearful that she has actually come to the movie alone. Believes everyone at work is playing a joke on her or knows something she doesn't. Has felt that people are taking her thoughts out of her head but not sure. Déjà vu—feels she has dreamt the clothes that people are wearing. Experiences never last for more than 15 minutes.

P1=6

Suspiciousness: Onset four years ago but worse in past two months.

Feels watched. Has felt as if someone in her house is waiting for her and occasionally when coming home will stay in her car until she feels "the coast is clear." She is not totally convinced but does not want to take a chance on being wrong. Feels people want her to fail. This is a general sense, no specifics and no delusional conviction.

P2=5

Grandiosity: Looks down on others as not as smart as he is, but keeps this private.

P3=1

Perceptual Abnormalities: Onset three years ago. Worse three months ago. Hears music or birds chirping inside at work when there is nothing. Hears people arguing or her brother's voice and looks around, but no one is there. Heard a brief scream while at work, it caused her to jump and no one else heard it. In total, two to five experiences per week for 5 to 10 seconds or so. Recently has seen people peeking out from behind a curtain of her house, and stayed in her car until her boyfriend came home. Once slept in her car. Usually can tell herself it is unlikely that there is someone there, but a few times thought it was likely and did not want to take the chance.

P4=5

Disorganized Communication: When tired or stressed (including interview) will go off track and need questions restated.

P5=2

Summary: Subject meets inclusion as a psychosis-risk subject with a 6 in P1 (very brief, up to 15 minutes). Does *not* meet psychosis criteria, however, since P1 is not disorganizing or dangerous and has not occurred at the required frequency or duration. Meets criteria as a Psychosis-Risk subject with **Brief Intermittent Psychotic States (BIPS)**.

Case 6

Subject ID: Ivan

DEMOGRAPHICS: Ivan is an 18-year-old white male who lives with his grandmother and his mother. He reports spending a lot of his time taking care of his mother, who has had a difficult course of schizophrenia over the last 10 years. He also has been a primary caretaker for his grandmother, who has breast cancer. He is an only child, and his father left the family years ago and currently lives across the country. Ivan lived with him for several months his first year of high school, but it did not work out for unclear reasons. He is currently a high school senior but did not have enough credits to graduate. He hopes to complete his education and then study audio engineering at a local community college. He does not identify having a support system. He has stopped participating in sports and music over the last year.

CHIEF COMPLAINT: Ivan was referred by a treating psychiatrist for bizarre behavior, increasing paranoia, and multiple somatic complaints such as, "There are cracks in my head." Ivan's grandmother reported noticing similarities in behavior to the patient's mother when she began to develop psychosis, including agitation, "spacing out," and isolative behaviors. Ivan's chief complaint was trouble concentrating, remembering, and thinking quickly.

PAST PSYCHIATRIC HISTORY: Ivan was on an inpatient psychiatric unit six months ago, diagnosed with Marijuana Abuse, Psychosis, NOS. The medical record reported the patient felt he had "cracks" in his head, displayed brief but clear auditory hallucinations, described paranoid delusions, and said that he felt safe on the unit and his symptoms "resolved overnight." No meds were prescribed, and he was discharged in 10 days.

PAST MEDICAL HISTORY: Musculoskeletal pain secondary to motor vehicle accident one month ago.

SUBSTANCE ABUSE HISTORY: Occasional alcohol use, two beers twice per month. History of heavy marijuana use two years ago. Ivan currently minimizes use, reports using about one time in last month, denies that it has been a problem. History of legal related marijuana charges and positive marijuana toxicology screen when he was referred for psychiatric evaluation. No other substance use.

FAMILY PSYCHIATRIC HISTORY: His mother was diagnosed with schizophrenia and has had multiple inpatient admissions and medication trials. She has a history of noncompliance and a chronic course of illness.

SCID: Marijuana Abuse

DIPD: No diagnosis.

Current/Highest GAF in Past Year: 45/60

SOPS Ratings Summary:

Questionable Level of Unusual Thought Content: Ivan reports some longstanding superstitions and occasionally finds special meaning in songs that he hears on the radio. He attributes it to coincidence. He is not able to comment on feeling like he had cracks in his head when he was admitted to the hospital because he does not remember making the statement or feeling that way. He is very preoccupied during the interview with somatic issues, and frequently has to get up and move around or stretch. This could be related to soreness from his car accident one month ago though the possibility of somatic delusions was considered while he was inpatient.

P1=1

Moderate Level of Suspiciousness: Ivan reports longstanding suspiciousness, and said he was taught to be this way. He reports he grew up having to watch his back, and generally does not trust people. He also reports family and friends have turned their back on him because of his mom's illness and now he can not trust them. Ivan was guarded during some parts of the interview.

P2=3

Absence of Grandiose Ideas.

P3=0

Mild Level of Perceptual Abnormalities: Ivan reports occasional experiences of thinking he smells cigarette smoke when no one else does. This happens every couple of weeks and is not bothersome. He also reports that something gets "triggered and heightened" when someone raises their voice and he does not like it.

P4=2

Absence of Disorganized Communication.

P5=0

Summary: Psychotic Disorder, Residual Phase. Individual does not meet criteria for being a psychosis-risk subject because of a past history of psychosis. The symptoms he presents are residual symptoms of psychosis.

Case 7

Subject ID: Justin

DEMOGRAPHICS: Justin is a 15-year-old Asian male who lives with his father, stepmother, and his two siblings. His parents separated when he was seven. He sees his mother about twice a year, and speaks to her regularly. He is in the 10th grade. He had been an A student and active in sports last year, but this year he began failing most of his courses, and he stopped going to school, which prompted his referral for evaluation.

CHIEF COMPLAINT: He reports a major lowering in his interests and motivation, which has led him to stop going to school. He complains that his motivation is continually getting worse. He has trouble getting up in the morning and often stays at home all day long.

PAST TREATMENT HISTORY: A psychologist he saw referred him to the psychosis-risk clinic. Justin has never been on medication, but is currently being prescribed Luvox 50 mg.

FAMILY HISTORY: Justin's mother has schizophrenia.

SUBSTANCE ABUSE HISTORY: None.

SCID: No disorders.

DIPD: No disorders.

Current/Highest GAF in Past Year: 50/85

SUMMARY OF SOPS RATINGS:

Unusual Thought Content: Justin reported "feeling different" beginning five months ago. He says he has begun to feel sad or mad for no reason at all. He is puzzled as to why he went from being a good student with good attendance to struggling to even get out of bed. Nightly, he experiences racing thoughts. About once per month, Justin reports that mundane things in his dreams will come true. After he has had a dream, he will wonder why he dreamt it, and what it may mean will happen. When questioned further about this, he deemed this process nothing more than a coincidence.

P1=1

Suspiciousness: No evidence of suspiciousness.

P2=0

Grandiosity: No evidence of grandiosity.

P3=0

Perceptual Abnormalities/Hallucinations: Moderate level. Starting at the beginning of this year and happening about once a month, he hears noises including banging and clicking and his name being called. He says he usually recognizes the voice as being his father's or his brother's voice, and stated that it is faint, like a whisper.

P4=3

Disorganized Communication: No evidence of disorganized communication.

P5=0

Social Anhedonia: Although Justin reported a slight decrease in the time he spends with friends, he is still socially active, seeing his friends a couple times per week.

N1=0

Decreased Ideational Richness: No evidence of decreased ideation.

N5=0

Psychosis-Risk State: Justin meets criteria for **Genetic Risk and Deterioration** psychosis-risk state based on having a positive family history and a 30% drop in his GAF score. Perceptual abnormalities (P4) meet risk severity level but not risk frequency level (occurring at an average frequency of at least once per week in the past month).

Case 8

Subject ID: Kevin

DEMOGRAPHICS: Kevin is a 15-year-old Caucasian male who lives with his stepmother, father, and older brother. He has just completed his freshman year of high school.

CHIEF COMPLAINT: He was referred to a local mental health clinic by his general practitioner for suspiciousness and unusual thought patterns.

FAMILY PSYCHIATRIC HISTORY: The participant's biological family history is negative for psychosis.

TREATMENT HISTORY: Kevin was treated for depressive symptoms and OCD one year ago with Luvox and Wellbutrin.

SCID: Patient met criteria for past major depressive episode and OCD. He also reports occasional marijuana use (i.e., once every three months for the past 18 months).

DIPD: Meets criteria for Schizotypal Personality Disorder.

Current/Highest GAF in Past Year: 47/47

SIPS ratings results:

P1. Unusual Thought Content:

The participant reports experiencing occasional déjà vu experiences within the last 18 months in which he "knows he's supposed to say something or do something because it's happened before," like he is following a script. Patient does not know how to account for the experiences and mostly believes they are real—his only doubt is that no one has yet explained the phenomenon of déjà vu, but he did not doubt his own personal experiences.

The participant also expressed concern that others can hear his thoughts; this experience is ongoing and has been occurring since four years ago. He states, "I have this big … paranoia about people reading my mind." He reports that this experience is currently more annoying than distressing and that he sometimes tries actively to suppress his thoughts if he has an "embarrassing" song stuck in his head or of he's thinking "something stupid." To suppress his thoughts, patient engages in a "shutting-up process" that usually takes about five minutes, in which the patient "fills his head with TV static noise." Minimal doubt was induced, although he had not even thought that an alternative explanation for his experience could be possible.

The patient also expressed concern about special messages that are conveyed on the television. Although the patient stated he does not believe the TV communicates directly with him, he does think that there is a code embedded in many Discovery/History Channel type documentaries, that "there is something there that needs to be found and rearranged." He reports having this experience every two to three months for the past three to four years. The patient thinks it is fun to try and uncover "the code."

P1=5 longstanding and stable

P2. Suspiciousness/Persecutory Ideas:

The patient reports that he is "paranoid," that he feels people are singling him out and watching him. At the same time he questions the veracity of his experiences. The participant feels mistrustful of most people and has felt this way for the last two years. He says that "once he started realizing what people in the world are like," it did not bother him to be suspicious of others—he reports liking it. The patient still maintains the vestiges of a strongly held belief from about two years ago that his bedroom window was actually a one-way mirror behind which his parents had installed a camera to watch him: he does not really believe this is happening, but he keeps his blinds closed just in case.

The patient also reports an overarching, vague feeling of being persecuted with occasional pieces of "evidence" supporting that feeling. He gave an example of being in a movie theater and thinking everyone was in on a plot to make him mad by inducing technical difficulties with the projector.

P2=4 longstanding and stable

P3. Grandiosity.

P3=0

P4. Perceptual Abnormalities:

The patient experiences a ringing in his ears when it is really quiet (he calls it a "blaring, loud silence") that "drives him crazy." This happens three times a year for a few minutes at a time and has been occurring since he was in elementary school.

P4=2 longstanding and stable

P5. Disorganized Communication:

The participant used odd, metaphorical phrases only when describing his OCD symptoms, saying that his counting rituals keep him "feeling square and whole as opposed to broken and jagged."

P5=1

Psychosis-Risk Diagnosis: Because his positive symptom ratings are longstanding and stable, Kevin meets SPD criteria. Other SIPS ratings that are pertinent to this diagnosis are:

N1. Social Anhedonia:

The patient states that he prefers to be alone and spends most of his free time on his own playing video games, reading, or playing guitar. He has a friend he describes as "close." However he only sees this person every two to four weeks (although they communicate daily via phone or instant messaging). The "close" friend will soon be moving out of state, but the patient is apathetic about this. The patient also described two other people as casual friends, but he has little social contact with these individuals.

N1=4

N3. Expression of Emotion:

The participant presented with a very flat affect and says he has been told by others that he has no feelings and no heart. On occasion, however, he smiled inappropriately when describing distressing experiences (e.g., past suicidal ideations) and unusual ideas. The interview flow was easily maintained despite this.

N3=3

N4. Experience of Emotions and Self:

The patient reports that it is very rare for him to experience positive emotion. He stated that he fluctuates between no emotion and anger with occasional experiences of other emotions such as sadness or happiness.

N4=4

Summary: The patient meets the following criteria for **Schizotypal Personality Disorder**, all longstanding.

- lack of close friends
- inappropriate and constricted affect
- suspiciousness
- ideas of reference
- odd beliefs

Case 9

Subject ID: Lillian

DEMOGRAPHICS: Lillian is a 21-year-old female in her third year of university, studying psychology, living with three housemates in an apartment, and working part-time. She was a state ward from age 12 to 19. She has contact with her biological family and her foster parents. She has been very involved in church activities since age 18.

CHIEF COMPLAINT: She is self-referred, wishing for therapy to make sure she has no unresolved issues related to her chaotic upbringing and to be monitored with respect to her positive family history of psychosis.

PAST TREATMENT HISTORY: She has had one supportive therapy session and has taken Effexor for anxiety for several years.

FAMILY HISTORY: Lillian's father and mother have both been diagnosed with schizophrenia, and both of her older brothers have as well. Both her mother and her oldest brother are in long-term hospitalizations.

SUBSTANCE ABUSE HISTORY: Lillian started drinking and using marijuana at age 14, also used ecstasy, Special K, codeine, and cocaine on occasion. Drug use stopped at age 17.

SCID: Past marijuana dependence, sustained full remission.

DIPD: Nil.

Current/Highest GAF in Past Year: 80/80

SOPS RATINGS:

P1. Unusual Thought Content:

P1=0

P2. Suspiciousness:

P2=0

P3. Grandiosity:

P3=0

P4. Perceptual Abnormalities/Hallucinations:

P4=0

P5. Disorganized Communication:

P5=0

N1. Social Anhedonia:

N1=0

N5. Decreased Ideational Richness:

N5=0

Psychosis-Risk State: Help-Seeking Control, despite a strong family history.

Case 10

Subject ID: Mickey

BACKGROUND AND PRESENTING INFORMATION: Mickey is a 12-year-old Caucasian male who is in public middle school. He is the youngest of two children and lives with his parents in very impoverished circumstances in an upper-middle-class town. Both of Mickey's parents work long hours in menial jobs and Mickey spends a good deal of time alone.

REFERRAL SOURCE: The patient was referred to the risk syndrome clinic by a school social worker who was familiar with the clinic through prior presentations by clinic staff at her school.

PAST PSYCHIATRIC HISTORY: The patient has been evaluated previously by a psychologist for obsessional and isolational behaviors that occurred only in the school setting. The evaluation concluded that the diagnostic picture was not clear. The psychologist ruled out autism, Asperger's Syndrome, Pervasive Developmental Disorder, and psychosis and stated that the patient did not meet criteria for any Axis I disorder. The psychologist concluded that further evaluation was necessary. The patient attended regular classes in school until two months ago, when he was granted special education services due to emotional problems. He is an A and B student. He received three sessions of counseling in the sixth grade for his behavioral problems in school.

CURRENT AND PAST SUBSTANCE USE: He reports no substance experimentation or use/abuse.

SIGNIFICANT DEVELOPMENTAL AND MEDICAL DETAILS: Mickey did experience some anoxia with a nuchal cord at birth and required one additional day in the hospital. Subsequent to that he seemed to meet all developmental expectations. The patient does not have any significant chronic illnesses.

MEDICATION HISTORY: The patient is not currently on any medications and does not have a past history of prescribed medications.

FAMILY HISTORY OF MENTAL/SUBSTANCE ABUSE DISORDERS: The family reports no history of mental illness.

OTHER DIAGNOSES: Mickey met SCID criteria for Specific Phobia, heights and insects. He did not meet criteria for any diagnosis on the DIPD.

Current/Highest GAF in Past Year: 43/51

SUMMARY OF SOPS RATINGS:

The patient reported a moderate level of unusual thought content/ delusional ideas. Mickey reports having very vivid déjà vu experiences at least six times a week. He is not particularly bothered by this but he says it began only four months ago and he often wonders why it happens. He thinks it is his mind playing tricks on him. He admits that he daydreams almost every minute of the day, usually about video games. He stated that he does not think he gets confused between what is real or what is imaginary but he does think about monsters a good deal of the time. He believes in monsters, has very specific theories about them, and takes precautions to protect himself from them. Although he does not see the monsters, he imagines that they wear weird wooden masks and their body is just exposed muscles. He also believes that the monsters emit a high-pitched scream and that light kills them. Because of this, he turns the lights on and off before he enters a room, even in the daytime. This began at the beginning of this month and happens at least a couple of times a week. He states that he knows the monsters are not real but he is afraid anyway. When asked for an explanation, he said that he is afraid of the dark and it is probably his imagination.

P1=3

The patient reported a **questionably present level of suspiciousness/ persecutory ideas.** He said he is self-conscious and worries that when people notice him they will laugh at him or make fun of him. He said he knows it is because he acted out in class in the past.

P2=1

The patient reported a **moderate level of perceptual abnormalities.** Beginning four months ago he started seeing a blurry, ghost like thing at the foot of his bed. He stated that it happens at least a couple of times a week. He said he knows it is not real but it worries him because it keeps happening. He also reported hearing "static" and ringing in his ears. This began on a daily basis at the same time. He said at times the "static" can almost sound like background voices. He explains this as one more example of his body and mind playing tricks on him.

P4=3

The patient reported **no symptoms and displayed no signs of disorganized communication.**

P5=0

The patient reported a **questionably present level of social anhedonia.** He has three close friends and enjoys spending time with them in and out of school, but is socially awkward with the other kids in his school.

N1=1

The patient reported a **mild level of reduced ideational richness.** Mickey reports that almost every day he has difficulty grasping the ideas that people are saying to him. He did well on the similarities and missed one of the proverbs.

Conclusion: Based on the above ratings for P1 and P4 and the fact that these symptoms started within the past year and occur at least once a week, Mickey meets criteria for the APS Psychosis-Risk Syndrome.

Case 11

Subject ID: Nat

DEMOGRAPHICS: Nat is a 16-year-old African American male who is in 10th grade at a local high school. He is an only child from a divorced family.

FAMILY HISTORY: His mother reports an extensive history of mental health issues in the family. She herself is treated for Bipolar Disorder with Psychotic Features and OCD. A maternal uncle is treated for Chronic Paranoid Schizophrenia, and the maternal grandmother is treated for Bipolar Disorder with psychotic features.

MEDICAL HISTORY: Mother reports that Nat was a high-risk pregnancy and she was put on bed rest at six months. She was being treated for severe asthma as well as depression. She was on 100 mg of steroids a day during the pregnancy and using inhalers on a daily basis. She was given a C-section in her eighth month and states that the baby was healthy at birth but did get many colds growing up. He is not on any medications.

SCHOOL HISTORY: He was in special education classes until the sixth grade, at which time he was kept back. After that, he was placed in mainstream classes and did fairly well, earning As, Bs, and Cs. Currently he does well in school, As and Bs, until he gets suspended for his temper outbursts and has to make up the work he missed. He has missed 20 days of school due to fighting and outbursts. He does not report having any close friends and clearly has difficulty getting along with his friends in school.

SUBSTANCE ABUSE HISTORY: He reports that he began smoking marijuana at age 14. At that time he was smoking every weekend. The last time he smoked was two months ago. He stopped because of the strange experiences he was having (see below). He reports drinking alcohol a couple of times this past year at parties with his friends from school.

SCID: Intermittent Explosive Disorder.

DIPD: Antisocial features.

Current/Highest GAF in Past Year: 50/55

SIPS/SOPS

P1. Unusual Thought Content/Delusional Ideas:

The patient reported feeling not in control of his own thoughts and ideas, especially when he loses his temper. As stated, he has been suspended for a total of 20 days this school year due to these outbursts. This happens almost exclusively at school. Nat and his mother both report that he has had only one outburst at home. The patient also reports that he senses the presence of his deceased grandparents trying to communicate with him. He stated that this began five months ago at the beginning of the school year and occurs at least once a week. It does not frighten him because he thinks it is his mind playing tricks on him to reassure him when he is going through a bad time. He knows it is not real and states it does not alter his behavior.

P1=3

P2. Suspiciousness/Persecutory Ideas:

The patient reported that he believes he is being singled out and watched. He stated that he has to pay close attention to what is going on around him and he has to watch his back because people might be intending to harm him. He said this happens about twice a week in school. He said this does not always lead to losing his temper but it does make him irritable. He said it began five months ago, he is not sure why it is happening and sometimes he questions its reality.

P2=4

P3. Grandiose Ideas:

The patient did not report or exhibit any signs or symptoms of grandiosity.

P3=0

P4. Perceptual Abnormalities/Hallucinations:

Nat reports hearing somebody talking in his head. This usually happens when he is at his father's house. He will think maybe somebody nearby is talking but when he looks there is nobody around. He says sometimes it is a male voice and sometimes it is a female voice. It started six years ago and has recently become worse, occurring at least once a week for the past three months. He stated that he wonders if it is his deceased grandparents talking to him. He stated it does not scare him but it is bothersome because it distracts him. He says sometimes he might go outside when this happens to check if someone is there. He also reported seeing a vague figure of his grandmother out of the corner of his eye. This also occurs about once a week but not at the same time as the voice. This began one year ago.

P4=4

P5. Disorganized Communication:

Nat reported having a difficult time getting to his point when telling his friends a story. This was not noted in the interview, however.

P5=1

Summary: Based on the ratings of P1, P2, and P4, the patient meets criteria for an APS Psychosis-Risk Syndrome. P1 and P2 have begun in the past year and occur weekly. P4 is longstanding but has gotten worse in the past year.

Case 12

Subject ID: Ormand

DEMOGRAPHICS: Ormand is an 18-year-old Caucasian high school senior who lives with his paternal grandmother who has been his guardian since age 11 (following several years of parental abuse and neglect). Both parents live in different states and there is little contact—none with father in eight years. He is an A/B student, has played football and baseball, and has a girlfriend. He was recently suspended from school for possession of marijuana, paraphernalia, and a concealed weapon (brass knuckles). He was admitted to a psychiatric inpatient unit for evaluation of possible psychosis. This unit sent him to the psychosis risk clinic for a second opinion.

PAST PSYCHIATRIC HISTORY: Ormand was involuntarily petitioned by his counselor for threatening behavior toward his teacher; he wanted to shoot her and throw her out the window. He spent four days on a psychiatric unit prior to SIPS evaluation. He was diagnosed with Depression NOS and prescribed Lexapro. He is currently followed as outpatient. He had prior treatment for several years at a community mental health center for depression, PTSD, oppositional defiant disorder, marijuana abuse, and ADHD (Ritalin). No prior treatment with antipsychotics. History of carving tattoos on his arms. History of legal problems since age 11 (marijuana, stealing). History of involvement with juvenile court, department of social services, placement in residential treatment houses.

PAST MEDICAL HISTORY: Broke his hand one month ago punching his truck during an argument with his girlfriend.

SUBSTANCE ABUSE HISTORY: Marijuana use since age 12, current use every other week. He has been a suspected dealer at school. He has been using alcohol for the last year up to twice per week, about five beers each time. He tried cocaine once two months ago. Tobacco user.

FAMILY PSYCHIATRIC HISTORY: Paternal grandmother recently diagnosed with bipolar disorder but not on medication. Father with history of substance abuse, suicide attempt at age 16, and self-mutilation. Mother with history of substance abuse.

SCID: Depression NOS; Marijuana Abuse

DIPD: Antisocial Personality Disorder

Current/highest GAF in Past Year: 50/65

SOPS Ratings Summary:

P1: Ormand reports recurrent experiences starting eight months ago of having interactions with people who might not be on earth. He describes it mostly as an evil spirit or demon that is trying to get him to do bad things such as hurt other people. He reports this mostly happens in his house, which he reports is haunted, but he can also experience "demon thoughts" in other places. Ormand reports sometimes at night he feels like he is surrounded by evil and it makes him have thoughts about torturing or killing people. He has conversations with "the spirit" often disputing its requests. He has been having recurrent, vivid nightmares about hurting his teachers, hanging them, and torturing others. When asked Ormand reports mostly believing the thoughts are his own and doubt can be induced. He does find it bothersome, however. He has not acted on the thoughts to hurt others though he does attribute some of his bad decision making, e.g., hanging out with a bad crowd, possibly to the evil spirits. Ormand describes such experiences as occurring several times weekly with a worsening intensity and frequency in the past two months. Of note, Ormand's grandmother and other family members who have lived in the home where he is living also believe it to be haunted, though they have never experienced "evil" encounters.

P1=5 Severe But Not Psychotic Level of Unusual Thought Content.

P2: The patient reports having thoughts that others are talking about him. This began three months ago when "I got a pretty girlfriend and they don't think I can handle it." He also reports unjustified mistrust of his girlfriend. Finally, Ormand reports feeling singled out and watched at school by the police and teachers. This is likely, as he has had recent troubles at school. (Of note, since the initial interview, girlfriend did break up with Ormand.) He also seemed guarded during the interview.

P2=3 Moderate Level of Suspiciousness.

P3: He thinks he has a 70% chance of becoming a famous country singer, rap artist, or athlete. He reports he can travel and meet someone famous and they can make this happen. He also reports he likes to pretend he has more money that he does and he leads people to believe he is rich. These beliefs began in the last year and occur weekly. Ormand also reports sometimes feeling like he has been chosen—he describes this as being chosen to be "bad" (to do evil or mean things), even though he does not want to be, in order to influence others to do bad things. He also reports feeling an unexplainable ability to make himself look bigger (e.g., heavier, taller, stronger) than other people so people will not mess with him. He reports people actually comment that he is "big and strong."

P3=3 Moderate Level of Grandiose Ideas.

P4: Patient reports seeing shadows in his room at night that he thinks may be ghosts or evil spirits. He tries to get into bed and turn over as fast as he can so he does not have to see them. He acknowledges that it could be the way the light is, or his eyes playing tricks on him. He reports first noticing this several years ago but it has worsened recently in frequency to several times per week, and he has found it more bothersome and a little scary. He also reports he has heard demon voices, but actually describes the voice as his own and that he talks for the demon. He reports hearing this mostly at night, but in the last month has heard it during class telling him to "walk out of class." He copes by focusing his attention on something by staring, or by trying to go to sleep.

P4=3 Moderate Level of Perceptual Abnormalities.

P5: He is often vague. He reports his girlfriend tells him he says random things that do not make any sense. This is not noticeable in the interview.

P5=1 Questionably Present Level of Disorganized Communication.

N1: Ormand reports being socially active—he often does not come home at night, but he is only able to name one close friend, and his girlfriend. His grandmother reports he has been much more withdrawn and isolative over the last two months.

N1=1 Questionably Present Level Social Anhedonia.

Summary: Individual meets criteria as an APS Psychosis-Risk subject based on P1, P2, P3, and P4. All have started or worsened in the past year, occur weekly, and doubt about the reality of his unusual thoughts can be induced.

Case 13

Subject ID: Penelope

IDENTIFYING INFORMATION: Patient is a 16-year-old, single, Caucasian female who is a high school sophomore and lives with her mother.

PSYCHIATRIC HISTORY: Patient was initially referred to the risk clinic three years ago based on symptoms consistent with the Attenuated Positive Symptom risk syndrome. She has been followed through the subsequent three-year period. Patient currently does not take medication and has not been prescribed medication since her initial baseline assessment. She reports that she has never tried illegal drugs, does not drink alcohol, and endorses no allergies or history of medical problems.

FAMILY HISTORY: Patient's biological father has schizophrenia and has experienced numerous extended hospitalizations. Patient reports having little contact with him.

SOCIAL FUNCTIONING: Patient currently prefers to be alone most of the time. This includes school acquaintances and some extended family members. Patient's mother stated that the patient's best friend told her that "everyone thinks you're a freak" and that she did not know why they were ever friends. Penelope also endorsed experiencing a significant level of anxiety related to social situations. Regarding patient's social development, mother indicated she thought patient was an "odd" child and had some traits others might find "annoying." No friends for over a year.

ROLE FUNCTIONING: Penelope reported having difficulty concentrating in class and mother reported that a couple of the patient's teachers had complained about her lack of attention in class (e.g., teachers have reported that patient "zones out" during lectures and asks questions that have already been answered repeatedly). Mother stated that patient's recent decline in school was not considered significant by school staff because she is still getting average grades.

Current/Highest GAF in Past Year: 44/54

SOPS Positive Symptoms Ratings.

P1. Unusual Thought Content:

Patient expressed an interest in witchcraft, and stated she once did a lot of research online in order to learn how to cast spells. Patient indicated that she tried to cast a spell on her peers in order to make her more popular. Patient no longer spends time thinking about witchcraft or casting spells, but currently believes if she invested more time into learning witchcraft, she might be able to cast spells.

Patient indicated she used to be preoccupied with "hidden messages" in lyrics of songs. Currently, she does not think about the messages in songs but she still thinks messages might be present in songs. Patient equivocated on whether she believes she "reads into" songs messages that may not be there, or whether she believes she actually finds hidden messages in the lyrics. She does, however, assert that she finds "answers" by listening to the radio. Patient reported believing if you think hard enough, the world will provide answers to you. The instances in which she has noticed messages have decreased, but her belief has not changed in intensity.

Patient expressed concern about a "shadow man," a vague figure she sees sometimes, who she sometimes worries can somehow harm her, but who cannot move through closed doors.

Patient reported that sometimes things seem to go faster than usual (occasionally one hour seems like one minute). She stated this happens once or twice a month.

Patient stated that her friends think some of her ideas are bizarre and strange, but she does not fully understand why they feel this way.

P1=3: Moderate severity, stable intensity, frequency, and duration over the past year.

P2. Suspiciousness:

The patient stated that she thinks she sees a vague, dark figure in her peripheral vision a few times a months (also see P1 and P4), usually at night, which she refers to as "shadow man." She explained that she believes shadow man is unlikely to be real, but she occasionally feels afraid that he will harm her in some way while she is sleeping, and so she makes sure to close her bedroom door at night to prevent him from entering. This thought is moderately distressing, and occurs less than weekly (two to three times/month).

Patient reported her acquaintances all hate her and she thinks they might "plot against" her at school. She stated some of her peers have spread rumors around school about her being "weird" so "everyone at school thinks she is a freak." She feels ostracized socially. Her level of confidence regarding this belief is high; however, it should be noted that her mother corroborates the explanation that individuals at patient's school have referred to her as strange and stopped socializing with her.

P2=3: Moderate severity, stable intensity and frequency over past year

P3. Grandiose Ideas:

Patient reported she believes she is smarter than most people and is destined to become "something." Patient also indicated she feels time is running out to reach her potential and she is worried that she will not reach her goals.

P3=2: Mild

P4. Perceptual Abnormalities:

Patient indicated that for the past three years she has been seeing "shadow man." This thought is moderately distressing, and occurs less than weekly (two to three times/month). Also see items P1 and P2. Patient also reported that in the past year she has been slightly more sensitive to sounds, but is not distracted by things being slightly louder.

P4=3: Moderate severity, stable intensity, frequency, and duration over past year.

P5. Disorganized Communication:

During the assessment, patient was sometimes tangential and occasionally got lost in the conversation. Patient asked examiner to reorient her to the topic being discussed a couple of times during the assessment.

P5=2: Mild severity

Schizotypal Personality Disorder criteria met.

Ideas of reference: P1=3, messages hidden in lyrics, books.
Odd beliefs or magical thinking: P1=3, ideas about magical spells.
Unusual perceptual experiences: P4=3, visual illusions, sensitivity to sound.
Suspiciousness or paranoid ideation: P2=3, others at school "plot against" her.
Lack of close friends: Friendships ended at least one year ago.
Excessive social anxiety: Patient endorsed, especially severe at school (related to P2).

Summary: Patient meets criteria for Schizotypal Personality Disorder. She also has a first-degree relative with schizophrenia, but her GAF drop over the past year does not reach 30%, so she does not meet criteria for Genetic Risk and Deterioration Risk Syndrome.

Chapter 13

Differential Diagnosis of the Psychosis-Risk Syndrome

Chapter 12 details prototypical cases of psychosis risk. In actual practice, such cases may not always stand out and be easily identifiable. Many of the signs and symptoms characterizing risk for psychosis are also seen in other psychiatric disorders. The baseline evaluation must be sufficient to ensure that the clinical picture being seen is actually one of psychosis risk and not one of another psychiatric state or disorder. This is called "differential diagnosis" or determining whether psychiatric syndromes other than the risk syndrome can account for the clinical presentation of the client under evaluation.

The mental states and disorders that may "mimic" or be mistaken for the psychosis-risk syndrome can be found among other Axis I and Axis II clinical constellations. The most thorough "differential diagnostic" assessment, therefore, would involve conducting structured interviews for both Axis I and Axis II DSM-IV disorders, e.g., with the SCID[66] or KSADS[69] (if age 10–14) for Axis I and DIPD[67] or SCID for Axis II. In actual practice, however, only a limited number of psychiatric states and/or disorders are likely to be confused with the risk syndrome, making lengthy and detailed structured assessments unnecessary. These "usual suspect" states and disorders, i.e., those most likely to mimic psychosis-risk symptoms and syndromes, are noted and described briefly below. Following these are four case vignettes of "other" disorders that can, at least intermittently, look like a psychosis-risk syndrome. For a more detailed elaboration please consult standard clinical diagnostic reference sources such as DSM-IV[48].

Major Depression Without and With Psychotic Features

Symptoms of reality distortion to a non-psychotic degree are common in major depression such as unrealistically negative appraisals of self-worth. Most psychosis-risk patients, however, do not meet full criteria for major depression, are more likely to complain of emotional lability and/or numbness than of depression, and present with reality distortions that are usually mood incongruent with depressive affect.

Mania Without and With Psychotic Features

Symptoms of reality distortion to a non-psychotic degree are also common in hypomania and mania (such as unrealistically positive appraisals of self-worth). For most psychosis-risk patients the qualifications noted above for depression apply here as well. The risk-syndrome mood change is typically mild and reality distortions are usually mood incongruent with manic euphoria or irritability.

Anxiety Disorders

Symptoms of reality distortion to a non-psychotic degree are common in anxiety disorders, such as unrealistically critical interpretations of other's opinions in social anxiety disorder, or unrealistic appraisals of dangers to one's own safety or the safety of others in panic disorder, or unrealistic appraisal of a threat to self in PTSD, or an unrealistic appraisal of the consequences of not obeying ritual demands in OCD. Such common anxiety-related reality distortions are not characteristic for a psychosis-risk syndrome. However, anxiety can be prominent in patients who meet risk-syndrome criteria, in which case both diagnoses may be given.

Substance Use Disorders

Substance use is common in many risk-syndrome patients, especially substances known to induce or enhance perceptual distortions, illusions, and hallucinations. When the "risk-syndrome" symptoms are strongly intertwined temporally with substance use episodes, substance-induced psychosis may be considered. However, DSM-IV suggests that if such symptoms occur after 30 days of sobriety, they are not likely to be substance related.

Schizotypal Personality Disorder

As already discussed, schizotypal personality traits are often present from an early age, and are more enduring and stable. The disorder can coexist with the psychosis-risk syndrome but the two conditions are usually distinguished by course. Symptoms in the risk syndrome are recent and progressive, not longstanding and static. Comorbidity between the two conditions, however, may occur.

Borderline Personality Disorder

An unstable sense of identity with shifting self-images and dissociative symptoms characterizes borderline personality disorder and often begins or exacerbates in adolescence. These symptoms, plus transient psychotic experiences, may suggest a risk syndrome diagnosis. For the BPD patient, in contrast to the risk-syndrome patient, these symptoms are usually associated with a relentless and chronic pattern of intense, unstable relationships, impulsivity, and self-mutilation.

Other Disorders

Other disorders that may account for or be comorbid with risk syndromes are Attention Deficit Hyperactivity Disorder (ADHD), Eating Disorders, or Pervasive Developmental Disorders such as Asperger's Syndrome.

Illustrative Cases

The following case vignettes illustrate some of the differential diagnostic disorders mentioned above.

Case 1

Major Depressive Disorder

DEMOGRAPHICS AND HISTORY: Quinn is a 20-year-old African-American male referred by his psychotherapist. He is currently enrolled as a full-time student in his second year at college. He is employed part-time in the college dining hall. He lives on campus in a dormitory with a roommate.

Quinn's first quarter went well and he received good grades. By the second quarter, however, Quinn began failing multiple classes (especially science) and reported feeling as if things around him were strange. He stated that his mood was poor, depressed, irritable, and he had been sleeping too much (more than nine hours a night) for about six months, often sleeping through classes. Since two months ago, however, he has had difficulty sleeping, getting four hours of sleep, typically between 6 am and 10 am. He denies any suicidal ideation, but would place himself in dangerous situations such as walking to the campus through a dangerous part of town. Since one year ago he has burned himself intentionally on more than one occasion. He experiences severe avolition with significant difficulty motivating himself to perform most tasks. He socializes with others, but has great difficulty with any true intimacy or close relationships.

REASON FOR REFERRAL: The subject was referred due to deterioration in functioning and the possible onset of perceptual problems. His major complaint was social anxiety and depression. He also stated that he thought he was "crazy."

MEDICAL HISTORY: Subject reports no medical problems.

PSYCHIATRIC HISTORY: Subject is not taking any medication. He began seeing a psychotherapist for treatment of depression and self-injury one month prior to referral. He has no previous psychiatric history.

SUBSTANCE USE HISTORY: Last year the subject had been using marijuana about once per week and drinking alcohol almost daily. He also experimented with ecstasy and amphetamines. He now reports having abstained from drugs for the past five months and drinks alcohol once a week, consuming approximately five or six beverages on these occasions.

FAMILY PSYCHIATRIC HISTORY: Subject reports a sister who may be depressed. He recalled an incident last year during which she called the suicide hotline. He did not know whether she was ever treated or diagnosed as a result of this incident.

SCID INTERVIEW RESULTS:

Axis I: Major Depressive Disorder, Alcohol Dependence.

Axis II: Deferred.

Axis V: 43.

CURRENT/HIGHEST GAF IN PAST YEAR: 43/50

SOPS Ratings.

P1. Unusual Thought Content/Delusional Ideas = 4, onset date = five months ago

Subject reports feeling as if things seem out of place, but he can't locate the source for these feelings. He frequently feels like he is imagining things and states that "sometimes things seem like a dream." Subject states he has frequent déjà vu, particularly when he is tired, but he is not distressed by this. He also endorses an overwhelming sense of guilt, feeling he is guilty for "something" but not being able to identify what it is. These feelings of guilt are distressful for the subject. He believes that others know he is "bad inside" and he sees this when they look at him, although he says there are times when he thinks he's making it up.

P2. Suspiciousness/Persecutory Ideas = 2

Subject reports that he is vigilant and mistrustful of others. He relates this sense of vigilance to his overwhelming sense of guilt and the need to protect others from himself.

P3. Grandiose Ideas = 0

P4. Perceptual Abnormalities/Hallucinations = 1

Subject states that he has on several occasions seen things out of the corner of his eye. He is unable to describe these things in any more detail than "maybe something moving."

P5. Disorganized Communication = 0

Summary:

Subject meets APS criteria for P1. However, these symptoms are better accounted for by the Axis I disorder of Major Depressive Disorder, which was diagnosed in the SCID interview. His reports of dreamlike thoughts, déjà vu experiences, and feelings of being bad, guilty, and toxic to others are all consistent with depersonalization and depressive ideation that are seen commonly with MDD.

Case 2

Bipolar Disorder

DEMOGRAPHICS AND HISTORY: Rebecca is a 20-year-old single female referred by her therapist of one month. She has been a student at a local community college for four months but is not currently attending classes. The subject lives with her family.

The subject began seeking treatment by a psychotherapist due to "problems functioning." Subject is now working with her third therapist since that time. Rebecca reported hearing voices, impaired memory, problems controlling her behaviors, and a sense that she is not real. Subject reported that she feels suspicious of others, so much so that she sleeps with a knife and will carry scissors or other sharp instruments with her for protection. Recently she has been sleeping only four hours per night and has gone through periods during which she has remained awake for several days at a time.

Subject reports feeling more irritable in the past two months, becoming angry and argumentative with others. Subject has also noted mild depression with some anxiety. She has also had difficulty completing tasks and focusing her attention. She reports that her thoughts are racing and she has difficulty concentrating. Subject is enrolled in college, but has been unable to complete classes due to the increase in the severity of her symptoms.

She reported that she has been hearing voices intermittently since two months ago. The first voice she heard called her name, which she initially believed was her younger sibling playing a joke on her. After learning that the sibling was not at home, she came to believe that she might be hallucinating and was distressed by this. Some of the voices whisper, some comment, and some talk with each other, according to subject. During the evaluation, subject's speech was rapid and often difficult to interrupt.

REASON FOR REFERRAL: Rebecca was referred by her third therapist due to her recent decline in functioning.

MEDICAL HISTORY: Rebecca has no medical complaints or history and takes no medication.

PSYCHIATRIC HISTORY: Subject has refused any medication. She started psychotherapy twice a week with her current therapist two months ago.

SUBSTANCE USE HISTORY: Subject denies any current or past substance or alcohol use.

FAMILY PSYCHIATRIC HISTORY: Her family history includes an aunt and a maternal cousin who have been diagnosed with bipolar disorder. Her father may also have bipolar symptoms, but has never been diagnosed with any specific type of psychiatric disorder.

SCID INTERVIEW RESULTS:
Axis I: Bipolar I-Mixed Mania/Depression.
Axis II: Deferred.

CURRENT/HIGHEST GAF IN PAST YEAR: 42/52

SOPS Ratings

P1. Unusual Thought Content/Delusional Ideas = 5. Onset date = one month ago.

Subject reports feeling like things are different, alien. She stated that her mother feels different, like a stranger. Subject reports feeling "unreal" at times, more at night than during the day. She believes her thoughts are being controlled, but not sure by whom or in what way exactly. Subject is distressed by these thoughts/ideas and experiences them daily. Doubt can be induced by asking if the experiences are real.

P2. Suspiciousness/Persecutory Ideas = 5. Onset date = one month ago.

Subject is highly suspicious of others. She is vigilant, mistrustful, and always worried about her safety. She sleeps with a knife under her pillow and carries a metal pen for protection. Subject feels as though others are watching her and some may wish to harm her (particularly worries at bus stops). She is unsure why she feels this way and can agree when asked that some of her fears might be unfounded.

P3. Grandiose Ideas = 5

Subject made several unsolicited statements about how "gifted" she is and that she is smarter than most people. She also stated that she is a great dancer and will be famous one day if she can manage to get "discovered."

P4. Perceptual Abnormalities/Hallucinations = 4. Onset date = one month ago.

Subject reports hearing voices a few times per week saying "hello" or commenting. Sometimes the voices will talk about her or make fun of her, sometimes whisper. Subject also reports seeing shadows on a daily basis and that she has been feeling a sense of pressure or pain, primarily on the side of her head. She is distressed by these experiences but maintains perspective and is aware that these are not real.

P5. Disorganized Communication = 5. Onset date = one month ago.

During the interview subject's speech was rapid and difficult to interpret. She had difficulty responding to questioning in a goal-directed manner, frequently going off track tangentially. Subject was able to be redirected through questioning. This type of speech is new for the subject (past month).

Summary:
Subject meets APS criteria for all five symptom domains. However, these symptoms are better accounted for by the diagnosis of Bipolar Disorder I-Mixed Affect type (mania and depression). All symptom domains were positive with four bordering on psychotic, and their present severity is new and of relatively recent onset (past month). The patient is in need of immediate therapeutic attention, including medication and/or hospitalization.

Case 3

Obsessive-Compulsive Disorder

DEMOGRAPHICS: Shawndriell is a 17-year-old African American female, and was referred by a psychologist for unusual recurrent fears. She recently completed the 11th grade. She reported that she had always earned As and Bs until six months ago, when she began getting Cs. The patient also reported that prior to ninth grade she was "outgoing and popular," but since then she feels socially awkward and only spends time with a few close friends on a weekly basis. She has been receiving individual supportive therapy with the referring psychologist and has been taking Prozac (60 mg/day) for the past year. Treatment has had little impact on the frequency of her fears, but they seem less intense. No first-degree family history of psychosis, however mother reported that her sister was diagnosed with a pervasive developmental disorder.

The patient reported a history of cannabis use beginning six months ago. She reported smoking daily until two months ago when she decided to stop in order to save her money. The symptoms described below preceded and persisted after her cannabis use but they did appear to be exacerbated when she used.

CURRENT/HIGHEST GAF IN PAST YEAR: 60/64

Positive Symptoms.

P1: Unusual thought content = 4, longstanding

The patient reported inappropriate guilt and unusual beliefs pertaining to fears of becoming bad and evil. She reported that beginning at the age of seven, she had a longstanding belief that there was a man on the other side of her bedroom door at night that could read her thoughts and make her into "something evil." She also reported that she would protect herself from him by repeatedly reciting prayers, listing the names of people who love her, and placing pillows on the side of her bed. She reported that this used to occur monthly throughout her childhood.

The belief about the man outside of her door went away as she grew up, but the fear of "becoming something evil and out of control in the future" persisted and now occurs about twice a week. She "knows logically that it probably won't happen," but she reported feeling increasingly anxious by the thought and in the past months has been having difficulty sleeping.

Shawndriell also reported that she uses rituals daily such as walking specifically on sidewalks and counting in patterns of 1-2-1 to "prevent bad things from happening," but she was unsure about what specific bad things would occur.

Lastly, the patient is convinced she is a "bad person," despite evidence to the contrary provided by family members and friends. She reported that she has been troubled by ideas and feelings of badness and guilt daily since about one and a half years ago.

P2: Suspiciousness = 2
The patient reported that she feels like people are always judging her and think they are better than her since beginning high school. She reported that she assumes that others are thinking negatively of her but that they do not necessarily intend harm.

P3: Grandiosity = 2
The patient reported believing she may have the potential to be "all powerful like the Devil" two times per week within the past month, but she did not report having these abilities and powers currently. She reported that she knows this is logically not possible, but worries that she could do "great harm to many people." She also reported that she has kept these fears mostly to herself.

P4: Perceptual Abnormalities = 0
The patient denied the presence of perceptual abnormalities.

P5: Disorganized Communication = 0
The patient did not exhibit nor report disorganized communication.

Summary:
The patient would meet criteria for the APS criteria based on P1 symptoms in the risk range if they were not so longstanding. However, these

symptoms are better accounted for as symptoms of Obsessive-Compulsive Disorder. OCD is characterized as recurrent and persistent thoughts, impulses, or images that are experienced as intrusive, inappropriate, and that generate high levels of anxiety and distress. The person recognizes these mental events as their own and tries to suppress them with compulsions, i.e., repetitive behaviors or mental acts (e.g., counting). Please see DSM-IV for diagnostic details.

Case 4

Bulimic Disorder

BACKGROUND AND PRESENTING INFORMATION: Tasha is a 15-year-old Caucasian female who resides with her adoptive mother, adoptive grandmother, and her adoptive brother. Both of her birth parents are diagnosed with Paranoid Schizophrenia. She was removed from her birth parents' home as an infant after it was reported that she was withdrawn, undernourished, and suffering from failure to thrive. She was placed in foster care soon after that. She is currently in the ninth grade at a local public school in advanced level courses. Traditionally she has been a straight A student.

PRESENTING COMPLAINT: The patient reported recent changes such as: weepy affect, grades slipping, difficulty concentrating, and lack of attention to her personal appearance. She reported to the school social worker that she was vomiting after eating, which led to her referral to the clinic.

PAST PSYCHIATRIC HISTORY: None.

CURRENT AND PAST SUBSTANCE USE: The patient reported no substance use or experimentation.

SIGNIFICANT MEDICAL HISTORY: None.

MEDICATION HISTORY: The patient is currently not taking any medications and has never been prescribed medication in the past.

FAMILY HISTORY OF MENTAL/SUBSTANCE ABUSE DISORDERS: Both of Tasha's biological parents are diagnosed with Chronic Paranoid Schizophrenia and treated with medication. Both parents have histories of numerous psychiatric hospitalizations.

OTHER DIAGNOSES: Tasha met criteria on the KSADS for bulimia.

SUMMARY OF RATINGS:

P1. Unusual Thought Content = 4

The patient reported a moderately severe level of unusual thought content/delusional ideas. All of these ideas reported revolve around her eating issues. She stated that sometimes when she eats she loses control, feels empty inside, and eats too fast and too much. She stated that she does not feel like she can control these binges. After the binges she feels bad about herself. This leads to her thinking that she deserves to vomit because she "messed up" and let people down. These intrusive thoughts have a moderate impact on her daily activities as they result in impaired concentration. She stated that she believes that she is not thin enough and that binging will make her obese, which leads to additional vomiting after eating normal amounts of food. She is 5'3" and weighs 110 pounds. This began about a year and a half ago and has been happening at about the same rate since then—several days a week.

P2. Suspiciousness/Persecutory Ideas = 2

The patient reported a questionably present level of suspiciousness/persecutory ideas. She reported that sometimes when she walks into the classroom the kids look at her and stop talking. This makes her wonder if they were talking about her. She said this happens when other kids walk in as well. She said it has been happening since she entered middle school, about two years and occurs about once every couple of weeks. She reports no increase in frequency.

P3. Grandiose Ideas = 0

The patient did not report any symptoms of grandiosity.

P4. Perceptual Abnormalities = 0

The patient did not report any symptoms of perceptual abnormalities.

P5. Disorganized Communication = 0

The patient did not exhibit or report and symptoms of disorganized communication.

Prodromal State:

Because all of the unusual thoughts reported by the patient are better accounted for by the Axis I diagnosis of Bulimia and are longstanding and stable, and no other positive symptoms meet risk(+) threshold, the patient does not meet criteria for any psychosis-risk syndrome.

Chapter 14

Psychosis-Risk Patients over Time

The psychosis-risk syndromes by definition are pluripotential mental states. They have their own syndromal presentations and attendant disabilities but they also represent sign and symptom constellations that are transitional to more severe and/or enduring clinical denouements.

Longitudinal studies of risk-syndrome samples, cited in Chapters 1 and 2, outline the major longitudinal trajectories of patients meeting SIPS risk-syndrome criteria. From the NAPLS risk-syndrome longitudinal study, the largest sample to date to be tracked over time, the following major longitudinal patterns emerged over a two-and-a-half-year period following initial (baseline) evaluation.[51] Approximately one-third of patients went on to "convert," i.e., to develop a DSM-IV psychotic disorder (56% schizophrenia spectrum psychosis, 34% other nonaffective psychoses, 10% psychotic affective psychoses). More undoubtedly converted to psychosis after two and a half years, but we have no data beyond this point.

What about those who do not convert to psychosis? We have not yet looked systematically at our group data from this perspective and so cannot offer quantitative estimates of the other clinical transitions among these patients. Nevertheless, based on several years of clinical experience we have seen the following longitudinal patterns most frequently:

1. Remission from at-risk symptoms states. Such patients may later experience a risk "relapse."

2. Remission from risk symptoms but remaining symptomatic and meeting some other DSM diagnostic category (ADHD, OCD, PTSD, PDD, BPD, Dysthymic Disorder, MDD, BI, etc.).
3. Retaining risk symptoms, which do not get better or worse. Over time such patients will often eventually meet criteria for STPD.

This chapter provides case vignettes of the most common transitions over time in our psychosis-risk clinic: conversion to psychosis (Upton, Victor, Whitney, Xiva), conversion to STPD (Yelena), conversion to non-psychotic bipolar disorder (Zane) in a patient who did not meet risk-syndrome criteria, remission from risk (Alan), and onset of a risk state in a help-seeking control (Bartolo).

Case 1

Patient ID: Upton

BACKGROUND INFORMATION: The patient is a 15-year-old, single, Asian male, adopted at birth, who lives with his adoptive parents and younger adopted sister. He and his family moved abroad while he was still an infant and returned to the United States eight years ago. He was educated in private schools abroad. He attended a private school here in the United States until last year, when he enrolled in public high school. Upton is currently a sophomore.

REFERRAL SOURCE: The patient was referred to the risk-syndrome research clinic by a local child psychiatrist.

PRESENTING ISSUE: The patient began hearing background whispering six months prior to evaluation, and this worsened markedly five months ago. He also became troubled by some unusual ideas and beliefs and began experiencing difficulty in school.

PAST PSYCHIATRIC HISTORY: The patient was diagnosed overseas with ADHD when he started kindergarten. He was treated with medication for the ADHD when he returned to the United States but he developed leg tics and the medication was stopped. The tics subsided, but his attention deficit continued, and the patient was prescribed 80 mg of Strattera for treatment of this.

CURRENT AND PAST SUBSTANCE USE: The patient did not report any substance experimentation or use or abuse.

SIGNIFICANT MEDICAL HISTORY: The patient reports that he wears corrective lenses for distance vision.

FAMILY HISTORY OF MENTAL/SUBSTANCE ABUSE DISORDERS: Upton was adopted at birth, and very little is known about his birth family.

OTHER DIAGNOSES: The patient met criteria for ADHD. He did not meet criteria on the DIPD for any Axis II disorder.

Summary of Ratings

The patient reported a **severe but not psychotic level of unusual thought content.** He reported that sometimes he thinks that events that happen are clues put there for him—a type of "foresight." He also thinks that sometimes people can hear his thoughts. Upton reports some unusual thoughts and beliefs about mythological "gods" looking out for him. For example, he is a very accomplished swimmer and competes on the high school swim team. Sometimes he thinks the Greek god Poseidon is in the water encouraging him. He also has some expansive beliefs about his ability to see at night and how this may be a "foreshadowing" that he could become a vampire. Upton's skepticism remains intact, and these beliefs do not usually affect his functioning. Most of these symptoms began in the last six weeks and occur several times a week.

P1=5

The patient reported **a mild level of suspiciousness**. He sometimes doubts people's intentions and worries about his safety. He could not identify a clear source of danger but referred to certain groups of kids in school who were the "bad" kind.

P2=2

The patient reported **a moderate level of grandiosity.** Upton reported notions of being unusually gifted in the area of swimming, having the "gift of Poseidon" and also, in games involving strategy, having the "gift of Athena." He also reports being able to see at night in the way that other people see in the daytime. His explanation for these abilities is that we are all better at some things than others. These beliefs all began in the last two months and occur a couple of times a week.

P3=3

The patient reported **a moderately severe level of perceptual abnormalities.** He reported that at times he hears whispering in the background. It sounds like more than one voice but he cannot make out what they are saying. He stated he knows that they are not real, but they are bothersome. He also hears ringing in his ears and he will do a reality check with the people around him to see if they hear it or not. He also reports seeing shadowy figures out of the corner of his eye. This occurs mostly at night. Again, he knows it is not real but does worry about the source of the experiences. All of this began six months ago, worsened last month, and occurs several times a week.

P4=4

The patient did not report or exhibit any signs or symptoms of **disorganized communication.** He reported a longstanding history of going off track for brief periods of time during conversations. This was noted on only one occasion during the interview.

Psychosis-Risk: Based on the rating for P1, P3, and P4, the patient meets criteria as an Attenuated Positive Symptom Psychosis-Risk Syndrome.

Follow-up Assessment:

The patient was followed for monthly visits per the clinical-research protocol. He was experiencing a steady increase in the intensity and frequency of his positive symptoms. Within three months of his initial assessment, his symptoms crossed the threshold to severe and psychotic. The patient began believing that he could see himself grow gills to aid in his swimming. He also believed his eyes grew another lid so that he could see better under water. He also described a sensation between his shoulder blades that he believed was the development of "wing" like muscles to help him swim. At the same time these symptoms were worsening, the patient was experiencing more and more success on the swim team. He believes, with delusional conviction, that this success occurred because of the gills, the lids, and the "wing" muscles.

In addition, the whispering in the background became clear voices—at least two—that talked to him about what he should or shouldn't do throughout the day. He stated clearly that he could not dismiss what the voices say and believed they were there to help him.

The patient was diagnosed as meeting the level of psychosis as determined by the Presence of Psychosis Scale in the SIPS. The patient was started on an atypical antipsychotic medication and referred to a psychiatrist for (outpatient) treatment. He continued to be monitored over time in our clinic.

Case 2

Patient ID: Victor

Victor is a 15-year-old, African-American male who is repeating the ninth grade at a local high school. He repeated the grade because he was school avoidant and was absent for too many days in the year. When present his grades have consistently been average to above average. He was referred to the clinic by a school nurse because of his avoidant behavior.

At the time of the SIPS evaluation, Victor reported feeling sad and down but denied any suicidal ideation. He described that something had changed about him, changed in the way he felt and thought. He stated that something was wrong with him that other people didn't see. He also reported having difficulty remembering things because of his preoccupation with his thoughts.

PAST HISTORY: His mother reported that she had a normal pregnancy and delivery. She said that Victor met developmental milestones on time. She said he is generally in good health. He had several sports (basketball)-related injuries but no major health concerns. He takes no medications and has no history of psychiatric treatment. The family history is positive for schizophrenia in the paternal grandmother and paternal uncle.

CURRENT ISSUES: Victor reported drinking to intoxication on several occasions with friends and experimenting with pot on several occasions. He said that since he does not hang out with friends or go to school any longer, he has not participated in these activities for at least three months.

P1. Unusual Thought Content=5, severe but not psychotic.
Victor reported many symptoms of UTC. He stated it felt like he did not have control of his thoughts or actions, that he sometimes thought people could hear what he was thinking. He said he didn't know how it happened and perhaps it was his imagination, but he did worry that people might exploit him this way. He also reported that sometimes he thinks the TV has a camera and is recording him. This happens about once a week and began within the past eight months. He says he knows it is his imagination but sometimes he has to shut the TV off anyway. He also reported some unusual ideas based on Ninja theories that he has studied. He reported believing in the power of the Japanese skeleton and how it guides him through life. Although he stated that he believes in this theory, the interviewer could induce skepticism, and Victor could

admit that it was probably just his imagination. Victor also stated that he was relieved to find that we were asking him the right questions and perhaps that meant we understood what was happening to him. He said it made him hopeful that we might be able to help him.

P2. Suspiciousness=5, severe but not psychotic.
Victor reported loosely organized beliefs about people's hostile intentions. He reported thinking that his friends were out to get him. He stated that they do not like him, they think negatively of him and want to harm him. He stated they don't trust him and he doesn't trust them. He stated at times he is even suspicious of his own family. Because of these feelings, he does not attend school or spend time with friends. He does still spend time with his family. Perspective could be elicited with questioning (e.g., Are you sure this is real?").

P3. Grandiose Ideas=1.
Victor expressed some private thoughts of being superior to his friends in strength and fighting talent.

P4. Perceptual Abnormalities=5, severe but not psychotic.
Victor reported that he began seeing shadows out of the corner of his eye about one and a half years ago. These shadows have now taken the form of a figure that he called the "Dark Lord." He said that 90% of the time it occurs he thinks it is real and external to himself. He said the other 10% of the time he knows it is his imagination. When it is not happening he thinks it is his eyes playing tricks on him. He also reported being hypersensitive to light and seeing black dots in front of his eyes. These events happen once to twice a week and have worsened in the past three months. He also reported hearing sounds inside his head that resemble voices in the background. No one else is around, so that is why he believes it is in his head, but he does think at times that he is hearing it with his ears. Sometimes it is troublesome and sometimes not. He also reported at times hearing his own thoughts as if they were being spoken outside his head. When asked how he explained this he stated that sometimes he thinks he looks too much into his brain.

P5. Disorganized Communication=0.
Victor did not report or exhibit any signs or symptoms of disorganized communication.

Based on the ratings of P1, P2, and P4, Victor met criteria for the Attenuated Positive Symptoms Psychosis-Risk Syndrome.

Follow-up Assessments:
The patient was followed with monthly visits at the clinic for nine months. He had returned to school at least intermittently and began

taking guitar lessons, which he appeared to enjoy. He was still struggling with the positive symptoms, which seemed to be increasing in frequency. He was given the SOPS repeated measure at each visit and provided with a structured interpersonal therapy. At the time of the nine-month visit, he stopped getting up in the morning, did not attend school, failed to keep up his personal hygiene, and became so frightened by his experiences that he could not sleep. He reported that he could now see the Japanese skeleton and it had given him new abilities to raise and lower his body temperature, alter gravity, and read people's minds. These abilities scared other people so much that he was afraid they would harm him. This fear caused him to isolate in his room. He would not leave the house for fear that someone would harm him. He was suspicious of the food he was being served and would not eat many of his meals. The noises in his head became clear-cut voices that would comment on his activities.

The patient met the Presence of Psychosis Scale Criteria, was diagnosed as psychotic, immediately started on antipsychotic medication, and referred for psychiatric treatment. Within two months there was a major improvement in his condition.

Case 3

Subject ID: Whitney

Whitney is an 18-year-old female who graduated from high school and is now working at an entry-level position with a local corporation. Traditionally she has been an excellent student and athlete, very social and popular with her peers. She lives at home with her parents and a sibling. Her parents became concerned because her behavior became erratic and she became very moody and irritable. They worried that she was losing interest in pursuing a meaningful career and in hobbies and interests that had once been important to her.

Whitney was adopted at six weeks of age. Her adoptive mother reports that Whitney's biological father had Chronic Paranoid Schizophrenia. They had no other information about her biological family.

Whitney addressed her parent's complaints by saying that they did not know what to expect from a teenager. She did not think that she was any different from her friends, just that her parents were clueless.

Whitney reported social drinking with her friends but not in excess. She also reported some marijuana use during her high school years but not in the past three months.

P1. Unusual Thought Content=4, moderately severe.
Whitney reported that sometimes she believes she can predict the future. She said that in the past she was just very good at reading people but now it is more than that. She gave an example of being able to predict exactly a scenario that would occur with her boyfriend and another female. She stated it might just be good intuition but she thought maybe there was more to it. She said it has really developed in the past four months and it occurs several times per week. She said she doesn't change her behavior because of it but she does wonder how much stronger it will become.

P2. Suspiciousness=4, moderately severe.
Whitney reported that she notices that other girls are always watching her very closely. She said she thinks they want to hurt her because she is so attractive and popular with males. She said it is probably just that they are jealous of her but at times she does think they intend to harm her. She stated that this thought began about five months ago and occurs almost daily.

P3. Grandiose Ideas=4, moderately severe.
Whitney expressed several ideas of a grandiose nature. She believes that she is a good luck charm. She said that when bad things are about to happen to her friends and she is present, the bad thing does not happen. She said she has been noticing this for about nine months but now it is occurring more frequently, about once a week. She also believes this is tied into the fact that God watches out for her and protects her in ways that He does not protect others. She also described episodes where she behaves without regard to painful consequences in terms of spending money because she has unrealistic beliefs about her wealth.

P4. Perceptual Abnormalities=1, questionably present.
Whitney reported occasional but noticeably heightened sensitivity to noise.

P5. Disorganized Communication=0.
Whitney did not report or exhibit any signs or symptoms of disorganized communication.
Based on the ratings of P1, P2, and P3, Whitney met criteria for the Attenuated Positive Symptoms Psychosis-Risk Syndrome.

Follow-up Assessment:
The patient was followed with monthly visits at the clinic for six months. She continued to work at her entry job and started calling out sick with more frequency. She would talk about going to college but would never make any attempt to actualize this. She continued to live

at home with her family but would fail to come home at night on more and more occasions. She was charging large amounts of money on her credit cards.

She was given the SOPS repeated measure at each visit and provided with structured interpersonal therapy. Within two months of the original SIPS assessment her rating scores had increased to 5s. She lost many of her friends because of her paranoia. In the sixth month, her grandiose delusions were influencing her behavior to the point that she was taking dangerous risks and had to be hospitalized. After many episodes of noncompliance with medication, she is now being effectively treated with risperdal and lithium. She is also actively engaged in individual and group psychosocial treatments.

Case 4

Subject ID: Xiva

Xiva is a 17-year-old Caucasian female who is in the 12th grade at a local high school. She was an A student until her junior year of high school, when her grades dropped to Bs and she began struggling with her school work. She began withdrawing from friends and family and lost interest in most things. She was referred to the clinic by her therapist, who became concerned that she was exhibiting symptoms beyond depression.

At the time of the SIPS evaluation, Xiva reported feeling an unpleasant mixture of depression, irritability, and anxiety. She also reported sensitivity to light and sound and some unusual perceptual experiences. She stated that she was different from other people and did not feel like herself anymore.

Her mother reported Xiva was the product of a normal pregnancy and delivery aided by forceps. She said that Xiva met developmental milestones on time, and she is generally in good health. The family history is positive for MDD with psychotic features in the maternal grandmother and Bipolar Disorder with Psychotic Features in a paternal uncle.

Xiva reported no experimentation or use of drugs and alcohol.

P1. Unusual Thought Content=3, moderate.
Xiva reported the occurrence of déjà vu about twice a week. She stated that they were foggy recollections that began about six weeks ago. They were disturbing because she did not understand why they started or why they continue, and why they were happening more and more

frequently. She also reported that around the same time she began to feel that her thoughts were being said out loud so that other people could hear them. She said she would look around to see if people were reacting to her thoughts and when they weren't she would think it was her mind playing tricks on her. She stated that this was worrisome and it was happening several times a week. Sometimes, about once a week, she gets the idea that people can just read her mind. She says that she knows this isn't true but she keeps thinking it anyway. This also began about six weeks ago.

P2. Suspiciousness=3, moderate.
Xiva reported believing that people are untrustworthy and say negative things about her behind her back. She said that she didn't believe that they would harm her but she did feel mistrustful of them. She couldn't remember when this started exactly, but she knew it began within the past three months and now occurred almost daily.

P3. Grandiose Ideas=0.
Xiva did not express or exhibit any signs or symptoms of grandiosity.

P4. Perceptual Abnormalities=3, moderate.
Xiva reported that she began seeing shadows and vague wispy figures out of the corner of her eye about three months ago, and it occurs about twice a week. She also reports a heightened sensitivity to light and sound. This began at about the same time and is troublesome to her, especially in the school setting. She said it interferes with her ability to do her work. In addition, at least one or two times a week she hears her name being called, and will check, and no one is there. These experiences all started about the same time and are worrisome because they do not stop.

P5. Disorganized Communication=0.
Xiva did not report or exhibit any signs or symptoms of disorganized communication.

Current/Highest GAF in Past Year: 60/75
Based on the ratings of P1, P2, and P4, Xiva met criteria for the Attenuated Positive Symptom Psychosis-Risk Syndrome.

Follow-up Assessment:
The patient was followed with monthly visits at the clinic for seven months. She continued to struggle with her schoolwork, and her grades declined to the point where she was failing several classes. She was given the SOPS repeated measure at each visit and provided with structured interpersonal therapy. Her suspiciousness increased at each visit until it reached a psychotic level of intensity at the seven-month visit.

At that time she would only eat food that was sealed in plastic because she feared that people were trying to poison her, including her own family. She could not sleep at night for fear that people were watching her. Her suspiciousness, especially, reached a psychotic level for sufficient time to meet POPS criteria for psychosis. She entered the rescue arm of the study and was treated with close monitoring, supportive psychotherapy, family meetings, and atypical antipsychotic medication until she was transitioned to a community provider.

Case 5

Patient ID: Yelena

Yelena is a 17-year-old white female. Her parents are divorced, and she and her brother and her mother live in the original family home. She was homeschooled until high school, when she entered a local private school. She had been an A student but is now getting Cs and an occasional A. She was referred to the clinic because she began showing up at school with safety pins pinned through the skin on the side of her nose. It was reported that she lost 25 pounds in two months because she wouldn't eat. Three months ago people noticed a severe change in her behavior; she wouldn't go to school and refused to leave her room.

Yelena's mother reported that she had a normal pregnancy and delivery with Yelena. The baby was born healthy and met all development milestones on time. Her general health has always been good. Yelena has no history of previous psychiatric treatment, has never taken medications, and has a family history positive for Paranoid Schizophrenia in a grandparent.

Yelena reported that she has never experimented with or used drugs, alcohol, or nicotine in her life.

Yelena reported that she was very afraid of being perceived as different or abnormal and was wary about doing the interview. When the interviewer explained to her that the questions in the interview were not designed especially for her but that everyone was asked the same questions, she became more comfortable. About a third of the way through the interview she actually stopped the interviewer because she was weepy. She said that she was so relieved to know that these experiences happened to enough people that we actually wrote them down as questions. Her stress level was reduced and she was able to complete the interview in a more relaxed manner.

P1. Unusual Thought Content=5, severe but not psychotic.
Yelena endorsed many symptoms of unusual thought content. She reported that within the last six months she has begun to have dreams that were premonitions of things to come. She said these things often came true. When asked if she believed they came true because she dreamed them, she admitted that perhaps it was just a coincidence. She also reported that she thinks she has telepathic abilities and might be able to read people's minds. She stated that it started last month but is more intense every day and she is very focused on it. Although she does believe in this ability she allowed for the possibility that it might be coincidence. She also reported that things happening around her have a special meaning just for her. She stated it was God's way of asking her to communicate with people because they can't communicate with Him the way He needs them to do. This began in the past six months and occurs two to three times a week.

P2. Suspiciousness=1, questionably present.
She reported that she occasionally believes the kids at school are questioning her motives. She said these were not her friends, but other people.

P3. Grandiose Ideas=4, moderately severe.
Yelena reported loosely organized beliefs of power. She believes that she can read people's minds, that she can read people's auras, and that she has telepathic powers. She also believes she was chosen by God for a special role as outlined above. These ideas all began or worsened in the past year and occur several times a week. She said they are worrisome because they make her different from everyone else.

P4. Perceptual Abnormalities=4, moderately severe.
Yelena reported she often hears people walking when no one is there. She stated that sometimes it feels like someone is brushing her hair when no one is there. She also reported that when she looks at a picture or a painting, she will see things in it that are not there. She also sees shadows out of the corner of her eye that appear to take the shape of a man or an animal and she described them as "dark." These things began happening within the last three months and occur three to four times a week. When asked how she accounted for these experiences she said she was not sure of the source but she found them "intriguing."

P5. Disorganized Communication=3, moderate.
The patient exhibited metaphorical over-elaborate speech, occasionally using incorrect words or speaking about irrelevant topics. She was unclear when this began, but it was clearly evident in the interview.

Current/Highest GAF in Past Year: 50/80
Based on the ratings of P1, P3, P4, and P5, the patient meets criteria as Attenuated Positive Symptom Psychosis-Risk Syndrome.

Follow-up Assessment:
The patient was followed on a monthly basis at the clinic for two years. We monitored her symptoms using the SOPS repeated measure and provide structured interpersonal therapy. She was able to return to school, perform well academically, hold a job, reestablish friendships, and develop a romantic relationship. At the time she left for college, she was deemed to meet criteria for Schizotypal Personality Disorder because there was no significant change in the intensity or frequency of her symptoms. Rather, these experiences were melded into her personality, became part of who she was, and did not cause a drastic decline in her functioning.

Case 6

Patient ID: Zane

DEMOGRAPHICS: Zane is a 20-year-old Caucasian male. He is currently a part-time student at a local community college and works part-time as well. He is single and resides with his family. He is close with his family and has a group of friends. He recently ended a relationship with a girlfriend of one year. He contacted the clinic in response to an online description of the clinic.

PAST PSYCHIATRIC HISTORY: Zane reports that he had an episode of MDD when he was a sophomore in high school. His parents took him to a psychiatrist and he was treated as an outpatient with Zoloft for eight months.

MEDICAL HISTORY: He reports no health concerns, no head injuries, hospitalizations, or operations. He reports no other history of prescribed medications.

FAMILY HISTORY: He reports no history of psychosis in either first- or second-degree relatives.

SUBSTANCE ABUSE HISTORY: He reports that he will drink wine on occasion if out to dinner or at a party with friends. He reports no history of drug abuse/dependence.

SIPS/SOPS

P1. Unusual Thought Content/Delusional Ideas

Zane reported that about four months ago he began feeling that things have a special meaning for him. As an example he stated that he noticed more and more cars on the road that are his favorite shade of blue. He isn't really sure what significance this has and he stated he knows it is just a coincidence, but he does enjoy seeing his favorite color. He said it is not at all distressing and it occurs every two weeks.

P1=2

P2. Suspiciousness

Zane did not report or exhibit any signs or symptoms of suspiciousness.

P2=0

P3. Grandiose Ideas

Zane did not report or exhibit any signs or symptoms of grandiosity.

P3=0

P4. Perceptual Abnormalities

Zane reported that beginning a few weeks ago he noticed some puzzling perceptual experiences, like reaching for the remote and it is not there, looking away for a second and then realizing it is there. He said it isn't really a big deal but it happened two or three times.

P4=2

P5. Disorganized Communication

Zane would briefly go off track once or twice during the interview. He stated that this just started happening in the past two weeks.

P5=2

Follow-up Assessment:

Zane was entered into the study as a help-seeking control. He was monitored on a monthly basis using the SOPS repeated measure. Five months after his baseline, he began having difficulty sleeping and he noticed his thoughts racing. The interviewer noticed he was speaking very fast on the phone and she had trouble following his conversation. Two days later she called to check in on him. He reported that he stayed up all night writing his thoughts down on Post-it notes and hanging them on his bedroom walls. He said he went over 36 hours without sleep and claimed he could not sleep because he had so much energy and so much that he had to write down. He was directed to the ER and he was hospitalized for a manic episode. He was diagnosed with Bipolar Disorder and began treatment with a psychiatrist, who initiated individual and family psychosocial interventions, and prescribed Depakote.

Case 7

Patient ID: Alan

Alan is a 13-year-old white male, the youngest of two boys in a two-parent family. He was referred to the clinic because he was truant from school for four months for no known reason. Previously, he had above average academic performance. Now he stays in the house all day, only leaving it if accompanied by his parents. He has stopped seeing friends, is very irritable, and throws temper tantrums at home. He expresses an intense and abnormal interest in motocross racing and spends a good deal of time fantasizing about being a famous racer. He denies any substance use or experimentation and is in good health. He takes no medications.

His mother reports that the pregnancy and delivery were normal and that he met developmental milestones on time. The family history is positive for depression but negative for psychosis.

P1. Unusual Thought Content = 3, moderate
He thinks his cousin can read his mind. He was concerned that the interviewer might be able to do so as well. The interviewer reassured him that she could not read his mind, and he appeared to accept that fact and was quite comfortable for the rest of the interview. When asked how he accounted for the mind reading, he said it is some kind of "magical" coincidence. He said it is becoming more worrisome and difficult to dismiss because it keeps happening. He also reported that he believes he has a race track in his head and the cars keep zooming around the track. He said it sometimes interferes with his concentration. He said it is probably just his imagination, but it continues to occur on a regular basis. All of these symptoms began within the last six months and occur at least once a week.

P2. Suspiciousness = 3, moderate
He expressed the sense that people cannot be trusted. He believes he must "watch his back" to protect himself. He is only comfortable leaving the house when accompanied by his parents. This began within the last four months and occurs on a daily basis.

P3. Grandiose Ideas = 2, Mild
He reported that he thinks he'll be a NASCAR driver one day and that he is already an excellent mechanic. This appeared to be the youthful expansiveness or boastfulness of an adolescent as opposed to a grandiose delusion. This also began with the past six months.

P4. Perceptual Abnormalities = 2, mild
He reported on occasion seeing shadows out of the corner of his eye or hearing an unexplained noise, like a clanking. He said this is not particularly worrisome and began within the past month.

P5. Disorganized Communication = 0
The patient did not report or exhibit any signs or symptoms of disorganized communication.

Current/Highest GAF in Past Year: 45/80
Based on the ratings of P1 and P2, the patient met criteria as Attenuated Positive Symptom Psychosis-Risk Syndrome.

Follow-up Assessment:
The patient was followed on a monthly basis at the clinic for three years. His symptoms were monitored using the SOPS repeated measure and provided structured interpersonal therapy. Eight months after baseline his symptoms remitted. He returned to school, graduated high school, and motorcycle mechanic school. He currently resides up north and remains in contact with the clinic via phone. He has had a steady girlfriend for two years and appears to be functioning quite well.

Case 8

Patient ID: Bartolo

DEMOGRAPHICS: The patient is a 20-year-old mixed-race male. He currently lives with his paternal grandparents. He attended a university for two years and left due to academic probation. He was last employed four months ago. He is currently enrolled in community college. He has a girlfriend and a few friends.

MEDICAL HISTORY: The patient reports no pregnancy or birth complications, and he met developmental milestones on time. He reports a history of back and knee problems and sports-induced asthma.

PAST PSYCHIATRIC HISTORY: The patient reported no previous psychiatric history. He has never taken or been prescribed psychiatric medications.

FAMILY HISTORY: The patient reports no known family history of mental illness.

SUBSTANCE ABUSE HISTORY: The patient reported that he started drinking alcohol at age 18 and that currently he drinks socially once every two weeks. He reports that he has never been drunk. He reported that he has experimented with marijuana on four different occasions since age 18.

SIPS/SOPS

P1. Unusual Thought Content/Delusional Ideas:
Bartolo has strong opinions about religion and politics. He stated that others find his beliefs in this area to be odd. He reported that he finds these beliefs to be compelling and they consume a lot of his time. He read about character personality traits from the *Dungeons and Dragons* game. He began to apply these traits, especially the "chaotic neutral" and "neutral evil," to himself in a magical way. He finds these compelling beliefs to be very meaningful.

P1= 3

P2. Suspiciousness/Persecutory Ideas:
Bartolo reported some doubts about feeling safe, although he could not identify a source of danger and did not seem troubled by it. He stated this happened once or twice a month in the last six months.

P2=2

P3. Grandiose Ideas:
Bartolo did admit upon questioning that he sees himself as having superior intelligence. He stated that he does not discuss this with other people and it doesn't influence his decisions or behavior.

P3=2

P4. Perceptual Abnormalities/Hallucinations:
Bartolo reported some mild sensitivity to light and sounds. He said it began about two months ago and is not distressing.

P4=1

P5. Disorganized Communication:
Bartolo did not report or exhibit any disorganized communication.

P5=0

Follow-up Assessment:
Bartolo was enrolled in the study as a help-seeking control. He was followed on a monthly basis with the SOPS repeated measure. Four months after his baseline, he reported that he was feeling very mistrustful of others and thought that people were acting hostile toward him. He said he thought people at school were talking about him in a negative way, and it made him uncomfortable. He said it happened several times a week. In addition, he reported that his sensitivity to sound had increased to the point where he would hear odd noises that were not

there, like banging or hissing or background noise that he described as "static-like." He said he found it very odd, and it was distressing because it would not go away and it happened several times a week.

At this point, Bartolo rated 3 on P2 (Suspiciousness) with a worsening in the past four months and occurring several times a week. He rated 3 on Perceptual Abnormalities with a worsening in the past four months and occurring several times a week. Based on this information, the patient met criteria for the Attenuated Positive Symptom Psychosis-Risk Syndrome. He continued in the study as a risk(+) patient.

Handling Conversion to Psychosis in Our Risk-Syndrome Clinic

Four of the cases above transitioned to psychosis by meeting the SIPS Presence of Psychosis Scale criteria. Essentially the patients' risk symptoms reached a level 6 for a specified period of time, or if their symptoms were creating a crisis of safety, no time period was required and psychosis was declared to be present.

All of our patients received appropriate treatment for psychosis upon reaching this level of psychopathology. At our psychosis-risk clinic, we regard the presence of untreated positive psychotic symptoms as a medical emergency, and we prescribe antipsychotic pharmacotherapy as the therapeutic sine qua non for such a mental state (in addition to our ongoing individual and family psychosocial work). Furthermore, we define "danger to self and others" broadly, meaning that psychosis not only may be lethal to life and limb but also permanently damaging to one's social network, reputation, and standing with family, friends, and employers. Psychotically irrational behaviors, especially if they are frightening or threatening, are a major source of social stigma and ostracism that can have lifelong consequences.

By following our risk-syndrome patients on a regular basis we have been able to see conversion unfold and to be with the patient and his or her family during the process. The clinic as a whole is alert to the weekly and sometimes daily developments of such individuals. Monitoring and psychosocial interactions are intensified to keep the patient in everyone's focus both at home and in the clinic. Threats to the alliance between the clinic and the patient/family are monitored carefully so that if and when psychosis supervenes, the transition to first-episode psychosis treatment is immediate and seamless.

Our clinical experience with this process (though not a part of any formal study) has been encouraging. In virtually every case, the transition to psychotic status and treatment has been straightforward and routine, with most patients not missing any time at work or school. A treatment alliance with patient and family was already in place, and adherence to treatment (including medication) has been consistent. With timely intervention we have not seen the all-too-frequent nightmares of forced hospitalization, suspended civil liberties, disrupted social networks, and reactive stigmatization because of bizarre social behaviors. In fact, by engaging potentially first-episode patients in their risk-syndrome phase, the possibilities for tertiary prevention appear to be substantially enhanced.

Chapter 15

Rating Baseline Cases for Practice

This is the final sample of cases on which to exercise what you have learned. The cases include samples of the following: APPS Psychosis-Risk Syndromes, Genetic Risk and Deterioration Psychosis-Risk Syndromes, Brief Intermittent Psychotic States, Schizotypal Personality Disorder, and Help-Seeking Controls with other disorders. Assessment summaries for each case are at the end of the chapter.

Case 1

Subject ID: Candace

DEMOGRAPHICS: Candace is a 20-year-old single Caucasian female. She is a full-time student in her junior year of college. This is her third school in as many years. Since arriving, she reports a sense of not fitting in, despite having a group of friends and being involved in campus activities.

CHIEF COMPLAINT: She called the psychosis-risk clinic after seeing an advertisement in the newspaper for the program. She reported experiencing increased coincidences, intuitions, a sixth sense, and a general sense of being on the "edge of breaking through" into the mystical powers of the universe.

PAST PSYCHIATRIC HISTORY: Candace reports an episode of depression in her freshman year of college, precipitated by the divorce of her parents and her father's withdrawal of support and contact. She was treated with trials of antidepressants, as well as psychotherapy. The antidepressants seemed not to help, but she returned to psychotherapy briefly last year during a time of stress.

PAST MEDICAL HISTORY: None.

SUBSTANCE ABUSE HISTORY: Drinks alcohol socially. Has tried marijuana in the past.

FAMILY PSYCHIATRIC HISTORY: Candace reports a mother, sister, and maternal aunt with depression.

Schizotypal Personality Disorder: Criteria not met

Current/Highest GAF in Past year: 80/80

SCID: Past history of Major Depression

DIPD: No Axis II disorder

SOPS Ratings Summary:

Candace reports an increasing interest in and study of New Age philosophies over the past year. She states that this came about when she stumbled upon a book in a used book store that led her to a new awareness and understanding of life. Since opening her mind to this way of thinking, she has noticed increasingly more coincidences/signs. For example, she went to her usual place to study but there was no free space, so she just started walking and looking for a place to study, when suddenly a door blew open, she went in and it was a place to study. She reports that she frequently sees her "lucky number" eight and takes this to be a sign that she is on the right path, moving in the right direction. She believes there is a connection between the conscious and the unconscious that allows her to be "intuitive" and at times to have a "sixth sense." For example, she will think about a friend and then that person will call her, or she will correctly predict little things like the color of the shirt her professor will wear, etc. These experiences have been happening almost daily for the past seven months.

She also reports that over the past six months when she is meditating, she will sometimes sense "a presence," which she thinks could be her "guardian angel or her spirit guide." This happens weekly.

She can at times see an aura (iridescent waves) around people and "read their emotional state." She occasionally thinks about the possibility that people/the world are two-dimensional, like a hologram. She explains that her grandmother was known to be psychic and wonders if she has inherited her gift. Candace acknowledges that she has become more preoccupied with this way of thinking, spending more time meditating, and has become less interested in school or other topics of discussion. She finds these experiences "weird/odd" and meaningful but states about once a week she will stop meditating because she becomes scared that she will "go too far into the unknown."

She reports longstanding feelings of being judged by others, feels she is different and that others tend to criticize/judge her for that. These thoughts are longstanding and have not changed recently.

She states that she feels her gift of intuition/sixth sense is a special ability. She does discuss this with friends but does not boast or brag.

She reports that over the past six months, a couple of times a month, she will hear unusual knocking sounds and has heard her name called on two occasions when no one else is around. She explains that this could be her "spirit guide" trying to get her attention. She reports that on two occasions over the past six months she has smelled gingerbread when no one else could.

She reports that she will occasionally go off track in conversation and feels that it is becoming more noticeable over the past year. Her speech was at times fast paced, requiring her to repeat herself, but no significant problems with understandability were noted.

Case 2

Subject ID: Darik

BACKGROUND AND PRESENTING INFORMATION: Darik is a 15-year-old African American male who is in the eighth grade. He lives with his paternal grandmother some of the time and with his girlfriend some of the time. He is one of four children, although all of the children do not reside together.

REFERRAL SOURCE: The patient was referred to the risk clinic by a child psychiatrist who is familiar with the PRIME clinic, and who was concerned for Darik after an MRI and EEG showed no explanation for his reports of blurry vision and feeling spaced out.

PAST PSYCHIATRIC HISTORY: The patient participates in an outpatient group at a local children's health center that is run by a nurse practitioner and supervised by the child psychiatrist. The initial presenting problem was extreme anxiety.

CURRENT AND PAST SUBSTANCE USE: Darik reported smoking pot twice about a year ago. This was a very negative experience for him and he is concerned that his current problems are due to that experience. He reports no other drug use or experimentation and reports that he drinks alcohol with friends on occasion, less than twice a month and never to the point of becoming intoxicated.

SIGNIFICANT DEVELOPMENTAL AND MEDICAL DETAILS: Darik's grandmother reports that his mother was addicted to crack and marijuana while pregnant with him. He was born premature at 35 weeks but still weighed over six pounds at birth, appeared fine, and did not need to be placed in an incubator. Most developmental milestones were reached on time. However, Darik was a late talker and his teeth did not come in until very late. Darik was hospitalized approximately six times during his lifetime for asthma/pneumonia-related illness. Darik has always attended regular classes in public school and is a B/C student. He was repeating the eighth grade because of significant absences last year.

EVALUATION: Darik was appropriately dressed, displayed a full range of affect, spoke clearly and directly, acknowledged having several close friends, and denied experiencing social anxiety.

MEDICATION HISTORY: Darik uses an albuterol inhaler to treat his asthma. He was tried on Seroquel for one week to treat his anxiety and sleep problems because the child psychiatrist suspected they might represent risk symptoms. He currently takes no psychiatric medications.

FAMILY HISTORY OF MENTAL/SUBSTANCE ABUSE DISORDERS: Both of Darik's parents are drug and alcohol dependent. His father is incarcerated. Two of his siblings are treated with psychiatric medications, both for anxiety and one for psychotic symptoms as well.

OTHER DIAGNOSES: Darik met DSM-IV lifetime criteria for Panic Disorder with Agoraphobia and Generalized Anxiety Disorder. Darik did not meet criteria for any personality disorder on the DIPD instrument, including Schizotypal Personality Disorder.

Current/Highest GAF in Past Year: 43/43

SUMMARY OF SIPS RATINGS:

Darik worries that something might be wrong with him like his brain is damaged from smoking pot. Despite reassurance from his doctor that there is no evidence to support this belief, it is still distressing to him. He describes feeling like he is "out of it," that he can't see well or hear well. This all began two years ago but is not getting worse. He reports that he daydreams a lot. He also reports that when he is out in public he feels like he is the center of people's attention. He does not think that people want to harm him, just that they all notice him more than other people. This also started two years ago and is not increasing in frequency. He also reports that he worries that his mind is playing tricks on him because he feels like things are moving in a "crazy" fashion. When asked to describe this he said it was like he couldn't tell if things were really happening or if it was his imagination. This began over a year ago and is occurring less frequently now.

Darik said he is self-conscious that when people notice him they will laugh at him or make fun of him. He does a reality check and realizes that they are not laughing, which calms him down.

Darik stated that he is a gifted rapper.

Beginning one and a half years ago Darik started seeing flashes out of the corner of his eye a couple of times a weeks. This scared him at first. However, he has adjusted to it and they are occurring less frequently now, approximately twice a month. He also has the sense that his hearing is off and he can't hear as clearly as before. He also reports blurry vision although this sounds as if it is part of his panic attacks.

Darik stated that he will go off track during conversations because he is a random thinker. He did ramble and go off track at times during the interview but responded to redirection. Both he and his grandmother reported that this has been a problem his whole life and is not worsening.

Darik has friends and a steady girlfriend and spends time with his family. He plays basketball and baseball. He states there are times when he feels uncomfortable or awkward around people and prefers to be alone.

Darik did exhibit some problem with grasping the meaning of the conversation. He did well with the similarities but had difficulty with the proverbs.

Case 3

Patient ID: Ethan

DEMOGRAPHICS: Ethan is an 18-year-old single Caucasian male who is a freshman in college. He lives in a dorm with a roommate and two suitemates. He did not do well academically his first semester and failed three classes. He has a good support system of friends, and supportive parents who live locally. They divorced when he was seven. He has no siblings. He comes home every weekend to work on his car.

CHIEF COMPLAINT: Ethan was referred by a university attending psychiatrist to the risk-syndrome clinic due to concerns about possible psychotic symptoms.

PAST PSYCHIATRIC HISTORY: For the past three months he has been seeing a therapist and a psychiatrist in student counseling services for depression and trouble with memory. He was started on Lexapro, which he still takes.

PAST MEDICAL HISTORY: None

SUBSTANCE ABUSE HISTORY: Occasional alcohol use, i.e., two times per month, not in excess. Rare use of marijuana, twice in the last seven months.

FAMILY PSYCHIATRIC HISTORY: Mother treated for depression; maternal grandfather treated with ECT for depression.

SCID: Major Depression, not in last month

DIPD: No personality disorders

Criteria for Schizotypal Personality Disorder: Not met.

Current/Highest GAF in Past Year: 65/78

SIPS Interview:

Ethan reports he began noticing coincidences about one year ago, and this has increased over the past six months to one to three times per week. These include light bulbs burning out or coming on when he walks by, thinking about a song which then plays even though his iPod is on random shuffle, and predicting what is going to happen next in a TV program. Ethan is uncertain about these coincidences and is puzzled by them. He has done some reality testing, like if he has song lyrics in his head and he is listening to the radio he will change the station to see if the song will play. He reports a feeling of connectedness with the music, but does not dwell on it. He finds these experiences unusual and does not think it is something he is causing but notes that it seems to be a relatively common occurrence. He also reports about once per month he becomes confused about dreams and reality. He reports that sometimes his dreams seem so real he has to ask friends to find out if they really happened or if he just dreamt it. This first occurred six months ago.

Ethan reports weekly incidents of unusual perceptual experiences beginning four months ago. He reports for about one or two seconds he will see a mouse run across the floor, or a black object fly across the window. When he double checks he does not see anything, and figures his eyes are playing tricks on him. He also describes experiencing repeated illusions, for example, when driving, he will think he sees a large black man with a white shirt and orange shorts walking. He also describes fleeting experiences of seeing a large black circle on his comforter that was not there, and seeing something on the TV that was not there. Both of these occurred when he was tired. He also describes an experience about once per month when his hands or feet feel detached after he has been sitting still for awhile (in a car, or in class). When this occurs he feels like his hands/feet are in a forest jungle during the dinosaur age. The only other way he is able to explain this is that it "feels old." Finally, he reports he is very sensitive to the hum of a television and can hear it far away when others do not notice it.

Ethan reports that in the last six months, about once every two weeks, he has noticed that he mixes up words in his sentences. For example, instead of saying "I put water in the beaker" he says, "I put beaker in the water." He also mixes up numbers on occasion. These are not noticed in the interview.

Case 4

Subject ID: Felipe

DEMOGRAPHICS: Felipe is a 21-year-old single male who lives in a fraternity house in town. He is finishing his second year of a nuclear engineering program and is currently working full-time at an automotive garage for the summer.

CHIEF COMPLAINT: Felipe disclosed that he was experiencing what he refers to as "schizophrenic symptoms" to his psychiatrist 11 months ago. The psychiatrist referred him to the risk-syndrome clinic. He also has longstanding difficulties with anxiety and flat mood.

PAST TREATMENT HISTORY: Felipe had been seeing this psychiatrist for approximately four years because of anxiety symptoms. He was diagnosed with OCD and panic disorder and was prescribed Effexor for this. A year later he disclosed that he was experiencing mild perceptual abnormalities and sleep difficulties, and his psychiatrist then prescribed 1 mg risperidone. Felipe took the medication for one week and missed many scheduled doses.

SUBSTANCE ABUSE HISTORY: Social alcohol and cannabis use.

SCID: OCD, Panic disorder without agoraphobia.

SOPS Ratings:

Felipe described a longstanding sense that something is "off" and things do not feel real. This occurs rarely and lasts for a few minutes. He also said that he occasionally has fleeting thoughts that someone can read his mind or that his thoughts are being said aloud, but these are easily dismissed and do not cause distress or cause him to change his behavior.

Felipe often feels that strangers think negatively of him and he is generally mistrustful. He describes being vigilant in public and worries about potential harm, but he does not feel that he is being targeted. He occasionally feels like he is being watched, but he is not sure who would do this or why they would single him out. He was guarded in the interview and was reluctant to have a student sit in on the assessment. He said he has been like this for as long as he can remember.

Felipe thinks of himself as highly intelligent and feels that he is more intelligent than many people, including some of his professors at school. He said that he enjoys debating with his professors and watching them become flustered. He did present with an attitude of superiority, but did not promote unrealistic plans.

For the past three years, Felipe has noticed that once or twice per month patterns will seem to be distorted and he will see spots across his visual field or he will briefly think he smells something that is not there such as flowers. These perceptual distortions do not impact his behavior, and he has no external attributions for the experience.

Felipe prefers to be alone but will participate passively in social activities with his fraternity brothers. He waits for others to initiate contact and says that he does not get much pleasure from socializing.

Case 5

Patient ID: Gina

BACKGROUND INFORMATION: Gina is a 16-year-old, single, Caucasian female who lives with her parents and two sisters. She is currently in the tenth grade in high school and is receiving Bs. This is a decline from previous years when she was a straight A student.

REFERRAL SOURCE: The patient was referred to the risk clinic by her mother, who is a psychologist for a local school and heard a presentation about the clinic.

PRESENTING ISSUE: The patient began complaining of an inability to sleep due to racing thoughts and severe nightmares, beginning within the past three months. Her grades have dropped, and she describes herself as very distracted. She reports feeling anxious around people but does have friends and is in involved in sports at school.

PAST PSYCHIATRIC HISTORY: The patient has never received psychiatric services in the past.

CURRENT AND PAST SUBSTANCE USE: The patient reports experimenting with pot two times in the past year. She also reports occasional alcohol consumption in social situations.

SIGNIFICANT MEDICAL HISTORY: The patient's mother reports that she had severe colic until she was six months old. This resulted in a failure to gain weight, not reaching 10 pounds until five and a half months old. One and one-half years ago she was diagnosed with ulcerative colitis. She has a history of some sports-related knee and shoulder injuries.

MEDICATION HISTORY: The patient was prescribed medication for her colitis.

FAMILY HISTORY OF MENTAL/SUBSTANCE ABUSE DISORDERS: There is a strong history of anxiety disorders on both sides of the family.

OTHER DIAGNOSES: The patient did not meet criteria for any Axis I or Axis II disorders.

Current/Highest GAF in past year: 60/90

Summary of Ratings:

The patient reported believing that things happening around her have a special meaning just for her. She will see something on TV and know that it is a message for her because of something she did. When people speak to her she believes it is God trying to send her a message because of something she did wrong or as a warning that something bad is going to happen. She said that these are occurring more frequently, every day now, and more intensely. She said she will avoid things or avoid saying certain things because of these messages. These beliefs are compelling, but the interviewer was able to induce doubt by eliciting her experiences of contrary evidence.

The patient reported that beginning three months ago she began to see vague, white, wispy figures out of the corner of her eye. She reported that she would turn to look and nothing would be there. She also reported that she would see movement out of the corner of her eye, something that looked like a cat or small animal, but nothing would be there. These incidents happen at least two to three times a week.

She also reported that at least one to two times a week she sees someone sitting in the rocking chair in her room. When she looks closely she realizes that no one is there. She said at the time it is happening the person appears very real to her. When questioned about it, she acknowledged that it could be her imagination. The patient also reported hearing sounds that no one else can hear. She said she will hear the garage door open and no one is there, or she will hear someone walking up the stairs and no one is there. She also hears a door slam or the TV turn on and there is no one there. These things happen almost daily. She worries that it is some psychic force trying to confuse her. She reports that these incidents are distressing to her and do frighten her at times. She will often keep the light on to help allay her fears. Again, upon questioning, she could admit that it might be her imagination.

Case 6

Subject ID: Heath

BACKGROUND INFORMATION: The patient is a 15-year-old Caucasian male who lives with his mother, stepfather, and his two siblings. His parents separated when the patient was seven, and he sees his father about twice a year, and speaks to him regularly. He is in the tenth grade and recently stopped going to school.

REFERRAL SOURCE: The patient was referred to the risk-syndrome clinic by a psychologist who saw Heath one time for evaluation due to school truancy.

PRESENTING ISSUE: The patient reports a major decrease in his mood and motivation, which has led him to stop attending school. He complains that both his mood and motivation are getting worse. Always mildly shy, he now spends no time with peers. He also isolates himself in his bedroom from family, seeing them only at meals.

PAST PSYCHIATRIC HISTORY: The patient saw a psychologist one time for an evaluation for the school.

CURRENT AND PAST SUBSTANCE USE: None reported.

SIGNIFICANT MEDICAL HISTORY: None reported.

MEDICATION HISTORY: The patient is currently being prescribed Luvox, 50 mg, by his primary care physician.

FAMILY HISTORY OF MENTAL/SUBSTANCE ABUSE DISORDERS: The patient's father is diagnosed and treated for Chronic Paranoid Schizophrenia.

OTHER DIAGNOSES: The patient did not meet criteria on the SCID for any Axis I Disorder and did not meet criteria on the DIPD for any Axis II Disorders.

Current/Highest GAF in Past Year: 40/60

Summary of Ratings:
The patient reported "feeling different" about three months ago. He says he has begun to feel sad or mad for no reason. He is puzzled as to why he went from being a good student with good attendance to struggling to even get out of bed. He reported no unusual thought content, suspiciousness, grandiosity, perceptual abnormalities, or problems communicating.

Case 7

Subject ID: Ingrid

BACKGROUND INFORMATION: The patient is a 20-year-old, single Caucasian female who just finished her sophomore year in college. During the school year she resides in the dorms at college and on school vacations and in the summer she lives at home with her parents and two younger siblings. The patient and her family report that she has been anxious and shy since the third grade.

REFERRAL SOURCE: The patient was referred to the risk-syndrome research clinic by her mother, who researched the clinic on the internet.

PRESENTING ISSUE: The patient reported difficulty with racing thoughts and thoughts that didn't make sense, some suspiciousness and some odd experiences with her hearing and vision.

PAST PSYCHIATRIC HISTORY: The patient first saw a doctor locally for treatment of social phobic anxiety in seventh grade. She was treated for this at the local children's center in ninth grade with CBT therapy and then began seeing a psychiatrist in 11th grade for medication.

CURRENT AND PAST SUBSTANCE USE: The patient reported no experimentation/use/abuse of any substances including alcohol.

SIGNIFICANT MEDICAL HISTORY: The patient was born three and a half weeks premature, but mother reports no difficulties at birth or immediately afterward. The patient met developmental milestones on time. The patient reported a history of recurrent abdominal discomfort from a very young age.

MEDICATION HISTORY: Patient reported being on Celexa two years ago. Last year it was changed to Zoloft and Xanax PRN because of anxiety. She reported that she does not have to use the Xanax once school ends for the summer.

FAMILY HISTORY OF MENTAL/SUBSTANCE ABUSE DISORDERS: The patient reported that both her maternal grandfather and grandmother suffered from anxiety disorders and were treated with medication. No other family history was reported.

OTHER DIAGNOSES: The patient met SCID criteria for Panic Disorder with Agoraphobia and Social Phobia. Based on the DIPD, the patient met criteria for Avoidant Personality Disorder and Dependent Personality Disorder. She did not meet criteria for Schizotypal Personality Disorder.

Summary of Ratings: The patient stated that six months ago she began having strange experiences. The first of these were very vivid déjà vu experiences on a daily basis, which led her to be confused about what was real and what was imaginary. She reported experiencing thoughts that were not her own that raced in her head, occurring about two times a week. She explained these experiences as her mind being "out of control" and playing tricks on her. She finds it worrisome now because it continues and will not stop. On a daily basis, she senses a presence in the bathroom when she is in the shower. When asked how she explains the presence she says that she thinks it may be an alien in there with her. She says logically she knows that it is not possible but at the time she does wonder about it. During the interview she expressed the concern that the interviewer could read her mind. She accepted the interviewer's assurance that she could not read her mind and continued to be open in her answers. She reported that such mind reading happens sometimes with her professors in school—approximately one time a week during the school year. She thinks this happens because she is very self-conscious about making a mistake or saying something stupid. Sometimes, however, she wonders whether it could be real.

She stated that on a daily basis she will think that people are laughing at her and talking about her. She quickly realizes it is not true but it continues to happen. This also began around six months ago. She stated that she also questions people's motives, i.e., why they are being friendly. When she received her grades for this semester, straight As, she thought someone was playing a joke on her and that they were not her true grades. She had to check the website several times to feel assured that they were indeed her real grades. She also expressed concern that her professors were watching her and singling her out from the other students. She said she did not like to think about these experiences and found them hard to talk about, but that they never went away. She seemed to be easily irritated by some of the questions during the interview.

The patient stated that she hears people in the house when no one is there. This occurs at least once a day and began when she returned home from school four months ago. She explains it as her "overactive" imagination. She reports hearing her own thoughts as if they are being spoken outside of her head. This occurs one to two times a week and began around two months ago. She is unsure what to make of this and wonders if it has something to do with her being too focused on her own thoughts. In addition, she experiences visual perceptual abnormalities, e.g., seeing shadows out of the corner of her eye at least once a day. This began about one year ago. She also thinks she sees someone out of the corner of her eye, about two times a week. She does a double take and realizes that no one is there. She said that she knows these experiences are not real, but she is unsure of the source, and they scare her.

The patient reported that she may briefly lose the point of what she is saying when telling stories or may get confused when trying to relate something to another person. This was noticed in the interview.

The patient reported having a very close friend whom she sees on a regular basis both during school and during the summer. Other than that friend she is not very social. Both she and her mother report that she used to be more social and was active in sports and dance. This changed during last summer. She does report preferring to be alone at times because she feels ill at ease with others, which is in keeping with her diagnosis of Social Phobia. She does spend time with family members on a regular basis.

Case 8

Subject ID: Jessie

DEMOGRAPHIC INFORMATION: Jessie is a 20-year-old single female recruited from an online notice at the college where she is a sophomore. She is unemployed and lives with her family.

REASON FOR REFERRAL: This subject reported a recent history of irritability, anger, poor sleep, and depressive symptoms. Her primary doctor thought this might be bipolar disorder but her psychiatrist diagnosed depression. She also reported a recent deterioration in functioning and paranoid thoughts. Her family history includes a maternal uncle who is bipolar, but no known first- or second-degree relatives with psychotic problems.

HPI: Subject reports that she has moments when she is fine, then has periods when she feels depressed, sad, or angry. These mood changes have been present for two years and last for a couple of days at a time. In the last two years, it has been extremely difficult for her to focus and study. She reported that she is easily distracted, has difficulty completing tasks, and is failing several classes. Subject's attention to hygiene has also declined in the last two years, now showering only once per week. She denies any history of insomnia but does at times have problems falling and staying asleep, feeling tired afterward. Her current medications include Prozac and a sleep medication. She has been treated intermittently since seventh grade by a therapist and psychiatrist due to fits of anger and depression. Past medications include sertraline and Lexapro.

On the SIPS interview, she reported that she sometimes gets suspicious, thinking that people think of her as a bad person and dislike her. These concerns have been present for the last year, especially about her neighbors, who she thinks watch her from their windows. These concerns about being watched are not a big bother to her, but she turns her shades so no one can look in. She reports that these worries have been a little worse lately and realizes it may be in her head although at times it seems very real. She does not change her behavior because of this but may isolate more.

She reports having had trouble trusting her family and classmates for years, and often believes that they are lying about small things. She prefers to be alone, can't stand being in public, and becomes preoccupied with the flaws of others.

She noted heightened sensitivity to sounds when she is trying to go to sleep. Her neighbors are very loud and at times she asks her mother if she hears them and she says no. This has been present for a while. She also endorses increased sensitivity to light that has been present since high school.

Recently she has found herself mixing words together, and going off track when she speaks. This is a new problem for her. This was not apparent in the interview.

On the SCID interview, subject also reported some obsessive traits, including hourly hand-washing, discomfort with things being out of place, and in the past has had obsessions about locking her front door four to five times per night.

TREATMENT HISTORY: Subject's primary care physician suggested that she may be bipolar, and her psychiatrist suggested depression. She is now taking Wellbutrin. She has taken Zoloft in the past but discontinued due to dizziness.

SUBSTANCE ABUSE HISTORY: Subject denies any substance or alcohol use.

DSM-IV DIAGNOSIS:

Axis I—Depressive Disorder NOS

Obsessive Compulsive Disorder

Axis II—Deferred

Case 9

Patient ID: Katherine

DEMOGRAPHICS: Katherine is a 30-year-old, single, Caucasian female who moved to her current home one year ago after living in the South for two years. She lives with her dog. She has an undergraduate degree and is taking online classes toward a master's in accounting. She has also taken online courses for an MBA degree. She does volunteer work with animals, and medically fragile elderly people, and is hoping to take an exam to become an accountant in the next few months. She has one friend here and tries to avoid contact with family in a neighboring state.

PAST PSYCHIATRIC HISTORY: No prior treatment

PAST MEDICAL HISTORY: Asthma; Allergies; Psoriasis

SUBSTANCE ABUSE HISTORY: None

FAMILY PSYCHIATRIC HISTORY: None reported

SCID: History of Major Depressive Episode five years ago. Treated with antidepressants for two years

Current/Highest GAF in Past Year: 68/75

SOPS Interview:

Katherine reports worsening experiences of "unreality" over the last year. She describes increasing confusion and puzzlement about what really happens or does not happen each day. This could be a simple thing such as whether or not she rang a doorbell at someone's house, or whether she had a particular conversation, or completed a particular piece of work. The experience usually lasts for a few seconds and she finds it bothersome. She is not sure what to attribute it to, but also reports many déjà vu experiences and wonders if it is part of that, or a lack of sleep. She also reports a sense that more is going on than she is aware of. She feels like it usually means something bad is going to happen but since she doesn't know what that is she is unable to prepare for it. She finds this worrisome and tries to focus herself by concentrating on the moment. This began two to three years ago but has been more frequent in the last year. She also describes some ideas of reference. She reports finding personal significance in certain state license plates, e.g., if she sees an Alabama plate and she is already anxious it means her anxiety will likely get worse, while seeing a plate from Ohio may bring her something good and is reassuring. She also finds significance in songs she hears on the radio. She reported being greatly moved when she heard our clinic's radio ad because she had been feeling lately like she was going crazy, and felt the ad may have been a joke. She reports that these experiences occur several times per week and have become more meaningful over the last year.

Katherine reports that for the last year, about twice a week, she gets the sense that strangers are watching her. She reports seeing people in places that are out of the ordinary and feels like they are taking notice of her and judging her. It makes her wonder if something is wrong. She reports this could happen anytime, like when she is walking her dog, or at the grocery store. She attributes it to "just me being paranoid." She also reports that over the last few months she will turn her work ID badge around so people cannot see who she is outside of the work place. She is not sure why, but guesses it is because she doesn't trust people.

In the last year she reports noticing smells others do not. She reports smelling unlikely things, such as lilacs in October. She reports for the last several months, about twice per week, she has noticed strange food smells in her apartment, or the smell of animal urine or feces. The way her apartment is situated it would be very unlikely that such smells would be coming in from somewhere else. She is not sure what to make of this and finds it strange and unsettling.

Katherine reports longstanding difficulty with word finding that has become more noticeable in conversations over the last year. It was not noticeable in the interview, although on several occasions she talked out loud to herself. She said she did not realize she was doing this.

Katherine reports a longstanding history of preferences to be alone. She spends most of her time with her dog. She is somewhat ill at ease around others and has minimal social interactions outside of work. She does have some old friends she communicates with through e-mail. She is not very involved with her family and did not feel comfortable discussing this during screening.

Case 10

Patient ID: Luke

The patient is a 14-year-old male who presented at the risk-syndrome clinic for an evaluation after being hospitalized for threatening to blow up the school and making threatening comments regarding his teachers. Luke had a very extensive collection of gypsy cards, and his parents took them from him because he was playing with the cards and not doing his school work. He states his father thinks the cards are evil spirits and threw them away. He blames his guidance counselor for telling his parents that he brought the cards to school. He states he has also considered damaging the counselor's office so he would know what it is like to lose something special. He states the cards are precious to him and there is no way to replace them.

The patient has no history of psychiatric treatment and reports no drug and alcohol use. He meets with his school counselor weekly for support due to poor grades and being picked on.

Current/Highest GAF in Past Year: 51/61

Interview:

Luke states he thinks he has an evil side or an evil spirit in him. He gave an example of opening the gate and allowing his uncle's two dogs to get away. He said his evil side opened the gate and let the dogs out. He states he doesn't remember opening the gate. He did acknowledge that it was possible someone else could have opened the gate since he didn't remember doing it. He states that the evil spirit is always messing around with his things. If he misplaces something he thinks it may be his evil side doing it. When asked by this interviewer if there may be another explanation he said it might also be his brothers. He said this started about five years ago and happens at least one or two times a week. He states he doesn't know what the evil spirit looks like. It could be a floating spirit or an animal. He states he heard it in his closet every night when he was trying to go to sleep. This began four years ago but he hasn't heard it in about three months.

Luke believes that people think he is too thin and will make comments toward him. He states even random people on the street will do this. He states he is being bullied at school. He doesn't trust people because they will take his things and lose them or use them without his permission. He states people often stare at him on the street and he thinks they want to take his bike.

Luke reports he hears his name called when he is in a crowd at school, the mall, or just walking on Main Street. It makes him angry, as he thinks it is someone actually calling him and not acknowledging it when he looks around. He feels it is disrespectful. This happens two times a week and began this school year, he is not exactly sure when.

He reported a one-time experience of thinking he saw a bird fly into the door. He was really perplexed because he looked for the bird and nothing was there.

He reports having an unpleasant smell of undetermined origin. He states it smells like poison. He thinks it could be the green mold that grows on wood. He states that if he thinks about the smell he smells it. He asks people if they smell it and it annoys him that he smells it and no one else can smell it. It can happen anywhere and he is absolutely sure that he smells it. It began just about a month ago and it bothers him a lot. He puts water or soap in his nose to make it go away. He smells the smell four times a week and it lasts for 30 minutes.

Luke's speech was circumstantial and he had difficulty getting to the point. His responses were often off topic because he perseverated a great deal about the loss of his cards. He reports he is a poor talker and sometimes doesn't know how to use the right words.

Case 11

Subject ID: Margarite

BACKGROUND INFORMATION: The patient is a 17-year-old single Hispanic female who is a junior in high school. Her parents divorced when she was a child. She lived with her mother and two brothers in Puerto Rico from age 3 to 11, when they returned to the United States. She continued to live with her mother and siblings until recently, when she moved in with her father. The change was made due to the increasing friction between her and her mother.

REFERRAL SOURCE: The patient was referred to the risk-syndrome research clinic by her father, who heard a presentation about the clinic at work.

PRESENTING ISSUE: The patient reported a decline in grades in school, a decline in her self-esteem, increased mood swings, trouble with focus and concentration, and social withdrawal. Her father reported seeing depression, irritability, mood swings, and impatience. Both reported that these changes had worsened since six months ago.

PAST PSYCHIATRIC HISTORY: The patient reported experiencing depression during the previous summer following the break-up with a boyfriend. She denied any other psychiatric history.

CURRENT AND PAST SUBSTANCE USE: The patient reported a recent history of marijuana use. She started smoking this year and smoked every day for one week. Since then she smokes about once a month and always in a social setting such as a party with friends. She says she has had sips of alcohol with meals in her home but does not drink in other settings.

SIGNIFICANT MEDICAL HISTORY: Father reported that the day after the patient was born she experienced a seizure. She was monitored in intensive care for two days. The cause of the seizure was never determined. Father reported that there has been no repeat of the seizure and no resulting problems from it.

MEDICATION HISTORY: Patient reported no history of medication use.

FAMILY HISTORY OF MENTAL/SUBSTANCE ABUSE DISORDERS: The patient reported that a grandparent was hospitalized many times during his life for episodes of bipolar disorder, that a grandmother is being treated with medication for depression and that an aunt is being treated with medication for schizophrenia. She denied other family history of psychiatric or substance abuse disorders.

OTHER DIAGNOSES: SCID findings revealed the following Axis I diagnoses:

296.25 Major Depression Disorder in Partial Remission.

The patient had met the diagnostic criteria for Major Depressive Disorder, single episode, moderate, one and a half years prior to this. Despite receiving no treatment, her symptoms moderated in two months and she no longer met full criteria for MDD. Since that time SCID findings support a diagnosis of MDD in partial remission.

Based on the DIPD-IV, the patient did not meet criteria for any Axis II disorders.

Current/Highest GAF in Past Year: 61/70

Evaluation:

Margarita stated that she occasionally wonders whether she has spoken her thoughts out loud without realizing it. She reported this experience mostly occurs when she is working out at a crowded gym while wearing headphones. However, on other occasions she stated that she will be deep in thought and think she spoke her thoughts out loud. She will do a reality check to see if anyone is looking at her. When asked whether she actually says her thoughts out loud unintentionally, she replied, "No, I don't actually do it. I just get this nagging feeling that I do." She stated that this experience is longstanding and happens approximately twice per month.

The patient stated that she occasionally thinks people might be looking at her in a negative way. She said she doesn't have a sense about who might actually do this, but just gets doubts about people's intentions toward her. This began this year and occurs twice a month.

The patient did not report any signs or symptoms of grandiosity.

The patient reported that on occasion she hears her name being called when no one is present, her cell ringing when it is not, and muffled noises when no one is around. She says these experiences are puzzling but she figures it is just her overactive imagination.

The patient denied communication difficulties and exhibited none during the interview.

Assessment Summaries

Candace meets an APS Psychosis-Risk Syndrome based on Unusual Thought Content (P1=3), Suspiciousness (P2=3), and Perceptual Abnormalities (P4=3). She also displayed a questionable level of Disorganized Communication (P5=1) and a mild level of Social Anhedonia (N1=2).

Darik did not meet criteria for a psychosis-risk syndrome. He was rated at a moderate level of Unusual Thought Content (P1=3) and a moderate level of Disorganized Communication (P5=3), but both of these symptom domains began over one year ago, have been long-standing, and were not getting worse. He did meet DSM-IV criteria for two disorders, Panic Disorder with Agoraphobia and Generalized Anxiety Disorder, which could account for some of his symptoms. As such Darik met criteria as a help-seeking control.

Ethan meets an Attenuated Positive Symptom (APS) Psychosis-Risk Syndrome based on Unusual Thought Content (P1=3) and Perceptual Abnormalities (P4=3).

Felipe did not meet criteria for a psychosis-risk syndrome. He scored at a moderately severe level of Suspiciousness (P2=4), a moderate level of Grandiosity (P3=3), and a moderate level of Perceptual Abnormalities (P4=3). All of these symptoms were longstanding, had begun prior to the past year, and were stable in intensity. Jesse met criteria for Schizotypal Personality Disorder.

Gina meets an APS Psychosis-Risk Syndrome based on Unusual Thought Content that is severe but not psychotic (P1=5) and on Perceptual Abnormalities that are also severe but not psychotic (P4=5).

Heath meets the Genetic Risk and Deterioration (GRD) Syndrome based on having a first-degree relative with psychosis and a GAF drop of more than 30% over the past year. He did not endorse any of the attenuated positive symptoms.

Ingrid meets an APS Psychosis-Risk Syndrome based on Unusual Thought Content (P1=4), Suspiciousness (P2=4), and Perceptual Abnormalities (P4=4). She also displayed a mild level of Disorganized Communication (P5=2) and a mild level of Social Anhedonia (N1=2).

Jessie meets APS criteria for P2. However, these symptoms are better accounted for by the Axis I disorder of Major Depressive Disorder, which was diagnosed in the SCID interview. Her concerns about being regarded as a bad person are consistent with ideation seen commonly in MDD.

Katherine meets an APS Psychosis-Risk Syndrome based on Unusual Thought Content (P1=4). She also displayed questionably present Suspiciousness (P2=1), mild Grandiose Ideas (P3=2), mild Perceptual Abnormalities (P4=2), and mild Disorganized Communication (P5=2).

Luke met criteria for Brief Intermittent Psychotic States (BIPS). He scored 5 on P1: Unusual Thought Content, 3 on P2: Suspiciousness/ Persecutory Ideas, and 4 on P5: Disorganized Communication. All of these symptoms were longstanding and established. The BIPS diagnosis comes from the rating of 6 on P4: Perceptual Abnormalities.

Margarita did not meet criteria for a psychosis-risk syndrome. She scored at the mild levels for Unusual Thought Content (P1=2), Suspiciousness (P2=2), and Perceptual Abnormalities (P4=2). She did meet DSM-IV criteria for Major Depression in partial remission. As such, Margarita met criteria as a help-seeking control.

PART C

The PRIME Clinic: Psychosis-Risk Patients Face-to-Face

Our clinical experiences over the past dozen-plus years with patients coming to the Yale University psychosis-risk clinic provide personal dressing to the numbers ultimately published as group statistics. Each of these numbers is a real individual struggling with the immense daily task of growing up, of negotiating the last major phase of neurological development that results in nature's most complex creation that we know of thus far, the adult brain of *Homo sapiens*.

Our patients illustrate, often painfully, that this developmental trajectory can suddenly and without warning swerve sideways from its expected, genetically programmed path. Sometimes this liability toward slippage is foreshadowed by developmentally earlier expressions of vulnerability such as childhood deficits in social or cognitive capacity or by early psychotic-like perceptual experiences, etc. However, the neurodevelopmental processes that lead to the majority of cases of psychotic disorder (e.g., aberrations in the management of synaptic pruning, as noted earlier) do not become biologically on line and active until adolescence.

Such timing, unfortunately, determines much of the chaos that commonly ensues. For most children entering adolescence, many developmental stages have already come and gone without problems, so very few in such families are looking for or expecting trouble. Thus, when the first signs of risk emerge, they almost always are met with disbelief and denial. The ones who cannot ignore the changes are the patients-to-be. Their minds suddenly, uncharacteristically cease to follow orders. Unusual thoughts, feelings, and sensory impressions invade their unique and formerly private conscious space and experience. Their minds no longer operate automatically as they used to. Sometimes their thinking even seems to be emerging from realms outside their own intention and control. They know something is very different, but they don't know what it is, how to describe it, or what to do about it.

Eventually their distress, disability, and helplessness becomes noticeable, and many (especially those from sensitive, intact families) find their way to the psychiatric healthcare system.

Management of Risk-Positive Patients in the Yale PRIME Clinic

PRIME is an acronym standing for Psychosis Risk Identification, Management, and Education. It identifies our psychosis-risk or "prodromal" clinic at the Yale University School of Medicine in New Haven, Connecticut. It was created in 1996 and has been located in psychiatric outpatient offices at two locations on the medical school campus, a smaller suite adjacent to a private academic psychiatric hospital and a larger suite located in the Connecticut Mental Health Center, a state-supported academic psychiatric treatment and teaching facility.

The staff consists of MD psychiatrists, PhD psychologists, MSW clinical practitioners, and trainees from all these disciplines. Professional staff are proficient in both clinical practice and research methodology. Most of the staff are actively engaged in clinical care and teaching in the medical school complex in addition to their commitments in the PRIME Clinic. The work of the clinic is supported largely by research grants, mostly from the National Institutes of Mental Health, but also from the pharmaceutical industry (for clinical trials of medication treatment) and from private donors (e.g., the Staglin Music Festival). In addition to conducting the studies for which the clinic has received funding, the tasks of the clinic include educating the potential referring community about the signs and symptoms of psychosis-risk and developing a network of clinicians and educators who refer potential at-risk candidates for evaluation at the clinic.

PRIME is at its core a medical-psychiatric center dedicated to the diagnosis, study, and treatment of patients who meet risk criteria for psychosis. Clientele always includes the patients, their families, and members of the referring network. It can also include key people from the patient's educational system.

Intake Evaluation

As described in more detail in Chapters 8–10, the intake evaluation of referred cases involves the candidate patient and his or her family. The candidate undergoes an extensive clinical evaluation centered around the SIPS and other diagnostic instruments, including structured interviews for Axis I and Axis II DSM-IV psychiatric disorders. Family members are usually involved, always if the patient is a minor. Past medical/psychiatric records are also collected and evaluated. Once the evaluation is complete, a meeting is set up with the patient and family to discuss evaluation results and to outline options. For patients who are risk(+), the clinic program and the (relevant) clinical studies are described. If they are interested they provide informed consent and are admitted to the clinic to start one or more of the protocols for which they have consented.

Standard PRIME Protocol and Treatment

Virtually all consenting patients are entered into an identical generic protocol of monitoring with the SIPS at periodic intervals. The intervals are monthly if the clinical picture is stable but may become more frequent if the clinical picture appears to be advancing in symptom frequency and clinical severity. The monitoring is usually done by persons on the team who also coordinate the patient's treatment and therefore are the most familiar with the patient's condition and that of the patient's family.

All patients in all studies are followed with the SIPS. All receive a generic treatment package in addition to SIPS monitoring. This consists of weekly individual supportive interpersonal therapy (SIT), which includes elements of psychoeducation (about risk, symptoms, psychosis, etc.) and cognitive behavioral therapy (about how to develop coping skills to deal with symptoms such as perceptual abnormalities).

Family meetings, with and without the patient, are established right away. One session of psychoeducation occurs early on with additional information supplied subsequently as needed. For all treatment studies families are offered individual therapy sessions, usually on a monthly basis. Contact with the family, of course, intensifies if ongoing crises demand more time and attention or the patient's symptomatic state begins to get worse.

Efforts are made to establish liaisons with each patient's school system (if they are minors). PRIME staff are available to consult with a patient's teacher or guidance counselor in order to apprise them of the patient's problem and his or her particular vulnerabilities (such as major problems with multitasking). Often teachers can structure classroom culture in ways that accommodate to the patient's problem with engagement and performing.

Medications for symptomatic anxiety and/or depression are allowed for most of the PRIME patients. Antipsychotic medication (or placebo) may also be given as part of a treatment study in which the patient has consented to participate. For example, this has included double-blind placebo-controlled clinical trials of Zyprexa, D-serine, and Geodon. Occasionally, patients will be followed in treatment by their own clinician outside of the PRIME Clinic. In such cases, the outside clinician may prescribe medication, including antipsychotic medication and PRIME research staff simply record what the patient has been receiving.

For risk(+) patients not in a treatment study and not being treated by a clinician outside of the PRIME Clinic, antipsychotic medications may be used by clinic staff in specified situations if deemed necessary. Clinical "necessity" is individually tailored but usually involves the evolution of one or more of the SIPS positive symptom scores to a level of 5. At such a juncture families are called in to discuss the situation and to be apprised as to what signs, symptoms, and behaviors would justify the use of antipsychotic medication. This could involve the escalation of any SIPS score to a level of 6 but could also include evidence of danger to self or others arising from a serious decline in functioning or reality testing.

Transition to Psychosis

As soon as the patient's mental state has reached a psychotic level of intensity and/or functional disability, he or she is started on antipsychotic medication by a PRIME Clinic psychiatrist. If a patient is in a treatment study, the antipsychotic medication prescribed will be the study medication. If the patient is not participating in such a study, the antipsychotic medication is chosen by the PRIME Clinic psychiatrist.

Patients are also evaluated as to the need for hospitalization, but this has seldom been an issue (see below). All other clinic therapies continue, and efforts begin to find an appropriate psychosis treatment team in the community to which the patient and family can be referred. We generally guarantee patient and family up to three months of continuing monitoring and treatment in the PRIME Clinic while appropriate treatment in the community is being sought. This includes medication coverage. Clinic staff can often be quite helpful in this process as they are quite familiar with the area treatment network, both public and private. They are also knowledgeable about special services available in the community for psychotic illness in youth such as therapeutic junior and senior high schools.

If the now first-episode psychotic patient is less than 18 years of age, he or she is referred to a child and adolescent psychiatrist. If over 18 years old, referral is made to an adult psychiatrist. Referral preference is given to psychiatric practices that include PhD, MSW, or APRN clinicians who are trained to provide psychosocial treatment modalities that complement the prescribed pharmacotherapy. Families with insurance are given a list of covered providers, including those with team practices. Families without insurance are set up with care structures of the State of Connecticut. This includes state insurance for minors and public mental healthcare centers for adults.

Other (False Positive) Transitions

Risk(+) patients not converting to psychosis make up the majority of PRIME Clinic patients. Four such cases are detailed in Chapter 13. As shown in Table C.1, among a sample of 81 patients diagnosed risk(+) and entering the PRIME protocol between 2003 and 2006, 61 or 75% did not convert to psychosis. Some of these went on to develop other DSM-IV disorders. For example (and not shown in the table), among the 33 nonconverting cases followed free of antipsychotic or protocol medication, 11 underwent follow-up SCID interviews and five of these had Axis I diagnoses that were not present at baseline: Major Depressive Disorder, Bipolar Disorder, Panic Disorder, Social Phobia, and Specific Phobia (one case each).

Among the same 33 untreated nonconverting cases, 25 returned for in-person follow-up SIPS evaluations. Of these, 11 remitted from their risk(+) symptoms (44% of the nonconverters). The majority of such remissions appeared to be spontaneous reversions to no disorder, thus suggesting that for them the risk syndrome was a clinical reflection of forces likely to be transitional/developmental in nature. The remainder (14/25, 56%) of the nonconverters continued to have risk(+) symptoms over available follow-up time, including three cases whose symptoms were sufficiently numerous and longstanding to meet criteria for emergent schizotypal personality disorder. The 44% rate of remission among nonconverters is to some degree an underestimate, due to the longer available follow-up time in the remitters (mean 21 months) than in the nonremitters (mean 9 months).

Table C.1 Psychosis-Risk Status and Conversion Yale University PRIME Clinic, 2003–2006

	N
SIPS Completed	222
Diagnosed risk(+)	96 (43%)
Open label studies of Abilify or glycine	7
Treated by community MDs with antipsychotics (Abilify, Risperdal, Seroquel)	8
Entered PRIME protocol	81
Number converting to psychotic disorders	20 (25%)
Schizophrenia	8
Schizoaffective Disorder	2
Bipolar Disorder with psychotic features	6
Psychosis NOS	3
Major Depressive Disorder with psychotic features	1
Converters receiving antipsychotic medication	20
Converters (also) requiring hospitalization	2

Risks and Benefits of Pre-Onset Detection and Intervention: Stigma versus Prevention

It has taken the healthcare system in America considerable time to realize the necessity for heightened vigilance during adolescence and young adulthood, and the importance of early detection for the prevention and treatment of "second neurodevelopmental phase onset disorders." The tardiness of such attention, in part, arises from resistance to identifying a potentially serious psychiatric disorder before it bursts forth on the scene in unmistakable form. The caution springs from a natural wish to avoid falsely declaring someone to be at risk, which currently happens two to three times as often as one "true positive" identification.

This conundrum of the relative burdens accruing to the true versus the false positive at-risk individual has elicited considerable debate within early-psychosis circles. Many see greater risks for those who are falsely identified and followed as risk-positive, their burden being the fear and stigma associated with the uncertain status of their health and sanity and their exposure to treatments that may not actually be necessary. These, indeed, are valid anxieties that must be anticipated and taken seriously. Nevertheless, stigma in our experience has not been a major issue because *all* persons coming to our clinic are help seeking. They come *because* they recognize that something is wrong, that a problem exists. They might not like that the problem is "psychiatric" but they have chosen to face their discomfort and the "stigma" of mental illness because of the nontrivial probability that such a malady may be on the near horizon.

The other reason stigma has not been a major impediment to participation is that the diagnosis is of risk, not disorder. Disorder is involved at this stage only as a probability. This state of uncertainty is discussed at length with patients and their families. Probabilities of disorder, if known, are shared, along with signs and symptoms that signal changes in level of risk. Analogies are made with other risk syndromes such as signs and symptoms of risk for diabetes or heart disease. Such information often helps to draw parallels with other, more familiar and less frightening disorders. Patients and their families become actively involved in tracking risk and in the process come to feel less helpless and victimized.

What about the true positives? The risks of not identifying and following those who are truly on a path toward psychosis are also far from trivial. They should hold considerable moral and medical weight as well. For "true positive" at risk persons, remaining silent exposes them to risks that we at PRIME consider to be far more substantial than those associated with false-positive cases. The consequences of ignoring risk, of not monitoring over time, of not being "ready," can be the bursting forth of an unexpected first psychotic break. Such an event is tragedy enough, but when it comes as a surprise to patient, family, and social network, the event can be chaotic and result in disaster. An unmonitored and untreated first psychotic "break" is a medical emergency in which irrational thinking and feeling can lead to behaviors that are highly destructive to physical safety, to social reputation, and to one's initial encounter and alliance with the treatment system.

At the very least psychosis-risk detection and monitoring over time can avoid such calamities. The survey of the outcomes of our PRIME Clinic referrals (summarized in Table C.1) illustrates this point. Over approximately two years of follow-up, 20 of the 81 patients in the PRIME protocol (25%) converted to psychosis. The conversion diagnoses are also listed in the table. This more recent rate of conversion to psychosis with medication-free follow-up is half of what we reported for a cohort enrolling in 1998–2000 (7/14 after one year, 50%)[50] and two-thirds of what we observed in our placebo control group enrolling in 1998–2003 (11/29 at one year, 38%).[29] The likely explanation for the differences is that in the early years, PRIME did not yet offer a structured monitoring program as an alternative to clinical trial participation. The availability of structured monitoring without medication seems to have attracted a population of patients who are at lower risk despite meeting criteria. The recent data also suggest, but of course do not prove, that risk syndrome patients who do elect to receive protocol or clinical medication may be at higher risk for psychosis to begin with and that the higher risk is then mitigated by the treatment.

All converters, per protocol, began receiving antipsychotic medication at conversion in addition to their ongoing psychosocial interventions. In only two cases was hospitalization necessary; one male became paranoid and frightened about his safety, and one female became suicidally depressed. Both managed to continue outpatient treatment after two and five days of hospitalization, respectively.

We feel these data support the thesis that early detection and monitoring of risk(+) individuals holds much more promise than risk for the future. In current practice it already achieves solid tertiary prevention, i.e., preventing the damage that can happen when an unexpected and unmonitored psychotic process erupts as a first-episode psychotic "break." Nine out of ten of our converters did not require hospitalization. In fact, most of them did not miss any work or school. They and their families were already in treatment, and the transition from risk(+) to psychosis(+) status and treatment occurred without any seismic "breaks" in the fabric of their lives.

Tertiary prevention is an obvious benefit of psychosis-risk identification and monitoring, but we also feel that detection and intervention in the risk phase of psychotic disorder has the potential of achieving even more powerful levels of prevention. Secondary prevention includes delaying the onset of psychosis, reducing the amount of time in active psychosis, and/or enhancing the treatability of the disorder. As noted in Chapter 1, early detection and intervention *after* onset, i.e., in the first episode phase of psychosis, can reduce the length and severity of that psychosis and preserve social and instrumental functional capacities. Given this, what more can be accomplished by identifying and treating the disorder at the time of onset, or even *before* onset in the risk(+) state? Currently, such benefits remain largely theoretical, and significantly more clinical research is required to demonstrate whether such potential can be realized. From our preliminary data, however, we contend that the benefits of risk(+) detection and intervention far outweigh the risks. Furthermore, we feel strongly that the time is at hand to undertake such investigations and for the criteria of the psychosis-risk syndrome to become a part of every diagnostic examination where such risk is suspected.

Bibliography

1. Rakfeldt, J., & McGlashan, T. H. (2001). Identification of vulnerable individuals before a first schizophrenic psychotic episode. In F. Flach (Ed.), *Directions in Psychiatry* (pp. 335–343). New York: The Hatherleigh Company.
2. McGlashan, T. H. (1984). The Chestnut Lodge follow-up study. II. Long-term outcome of schizophrenia and the affective disorders. *Archives of General Psychiatry*, 41(6), 586–601.
3. McGlashan, T. H. (1988). A selective review of recent North American long-term follow-up studies of schizophrenia. *Schizophrenia Bulletin*, 14(4), 515–542.
4. Jablensky, A., Sartorius, N., Ernberg, G., Anker, M., Korten, A., Cooper, J. E., et al. (1992). Schizophrenia: Manifestations, incidence, and course in different cultures. A World Health Organization ten-country study. [erratum appears in *Psychol Med Monogr Suppl* 1992 Nov;22(4): following 1092]. *Psychological Medicine—Monograph Supplement*, 20, 1–97.
5. Hafner, H., & an der Heiden, W. (1997). Epidemiology of schizophrenia *Canadian Journal of Psychiatry—Revue Canadienne de Psychiatrie*, 42(2), 139–151.
6. Kraepelin, E. (1971). *Dementia Praecox and Paraphrenia* [1919] (R. M. Barclay, Trans.). New York: Robert E. Krieger.
7. Wu, E.Q., Birnbaum, H.G., Shi, L., Ball, D.E., Kessler, R.C., Moulis, M., Aggarwal, M.H.S. (2005). The economic burden of schizophrenia in the United States. *Journal of Clinical Psychiatry*, 66, 1122–1129.
8. McGlashan, T. H. (1996). Early detection and intervention in schizophrenia: Editor's introduction. *Schizophrenia Bulletin*, 22(2), 197–199.

9. McGlashan, T. H., & Fenton, W. S. (1993). Subtype progression and pathophysiologic deterioration in early schizophrenia. *Schizophrenia Bulletin*, 19(1), 71–84.
10. Fenton, W. S., & McGlashan, T. H. (1994). Antecedents, symptom progression, and long-term outcome of the deficit syndrome in schizophrenia. *American Journal of Psychiatry*, 151(3), 351–356.
11. Tully, E., & McGlashan, T. H. (2006). The prodrome. In J. A. Lieberman & T. S. Stroup (Eds.), *Textbook of Schizophrenia* (pp. 341–352): American Psychiatric Publishing.
12. Beiser, M., Erickson, D., Fleming, J. A., & Iacono, W. G. (1993). Establishing the onset of psychotic illness. *American Journal of Psychiatry*, 150(9), 1349–1354.
13. McGlashan, T. H., & Hoffman, R. E. (2000). Schizophrenia as a disorder of developmentally reduced synaptic connectivity. *Archives of General Psychiatry*, 57(7), 637–648.
14. Susser, E., Neugebauer, R., Hoek, H. W., Brown, A. S., Lin, S., Labovitz, D., et al. (1996). Schizophrenia after prenatal famine. *Archives of General Psychiatry*, 53, 25–31.
15. Opjordsmoen, S. (1991). Long-term clinical outcome of schizophrenia with special reference to gender differences. *Acta Psychiatrica Scandinavica*, 83(4), 307–313.
16. Wyatt, R. J. (1991). Neuroleptics and the natural course of schizophrenia. *Schizophrenia Bulletin*, 17(2), 325–351.
17. Marshall, M., Lewis, S., Lockwood, A., Drake, R., Jones, P., & Croudace, T. (2005). Association between duration of untreated psychosis and outcome in cohorts of first-episode patients: A systematic review. *Archives of General Psychiatry*, 62(9), 975–983.
18. Perkins, D. O., Gu, H., Boteva, K., & Lieberman, J. A. (2005). Relationship between duration of untreated psychosis and outcome in first-episode schizophrenia: A critical review and meta-analysis. *American Journal of Psychiatry*, 162(10), 1785–1804.
19. McGlashan, T. H., & Johannessen, J. O. (1996). Early detection and intervention with schizophrenia: rationale. *Schizophrenia Bulletin*, 22(2), 201–222.
20. McGlashan, T. H. (1996). Early detection and intervention in schizophrenia: Research. *Schizophrenia Bulletin*, 22(2), 327–345.
21. Johannessen, J. O., McGlashan, T. H., Larsen, T. K., Horneland, M., Joa, I., Mardal, S., et al. (2001). Early detection strategies for untreated first-episode psychosis. *Schizophrenia Research*, 51(1), 39–46.
22. Larsen, T. K., McGlashan, T. H., Johannessen, J. O., Friis, S., Guldberg, C., Haahr, U., et al. (2001). Shortened duration of untreated first episode of psychosis: Changes in patient characteristics at treatment. *American Journal of Psychiatry*, 158:1917–1919.
23. Johannessen, J. O., Larsen, T. K., Horneland, M., Joa, I., Mardal, S., Kvebaek, R., et al. (2001). The TIPS project: A systematized program to reduce duration of untreated psychosis in first episode schizophrenia. In T. Miller et al. (Eds.), *Early Intervention in Psychotic Disorders* (pp. 151–166). The Netherlands: Kluwer Academic Publishers.
24. Melle, I., Larsen, T. K., Haahr, U., Friis, S., Johannessen, J. O., Opjordsmoen, S., et al. (2004). Reducing the duration of untreated first-episode psychosis: Effects on clinical presentation. *Archives of General Psychiatry*, 61(2), 143–150.
25. Melle, I., Johannesen, J. O., Friis, S., Haahr, U., Joa, I., Larsen, T. K., et al. (2006). Early detection of the first episode of schizophrenia and suicidal behavior. *American Journal of Psychiatry*, 163(5), 800–804.

26. Larsen, T. K., Melle, I., Auestad, B., Friis, S., Haahr, U., Johannessen, J. O., et al. (2006). Early detection of first-episode psychosis: The effect on one-year outcome. *Schizophrenia Bulletin*, 32(4), 758–764.
27. Melle, I., Larsen, T. K., Haahr, U., Friis, S., Johannesen, J. O., Opjordsmoen, S., et al. (2008). Prevention of negative symptom psychopathologies in first-episode schizophrenia: Two-year effects of reducing the duration of untreated psychosis. *Archives of General Psychiatry*, 65(6), 634–640.
28. McGorry, P. D., Yung, A. R., Phillips, L. J., Yuen, H. P., Francey, S., Cosgrave, E. M., et al. (2002). Randomized controlled trial of interventions designed to reduce the risk of progression to first-episode psychosis in a clinical sample with subthreshold symptoms. *Archives of General Psychiatry*, 59(10), 921–928.
29. McGlashan, T. H., Zipursky, R. B., Perkins, D., Addington, J., Miller, T., Woods, S. W., et al. (2006). Randomized, double-blind trial of olanzapine versus placebo in patients prodromally symptomatic for psychosis. *American Journal of Psychiatry*, 163(5), 790–799.
30. Morrison, A. P., French, P., Walford, L., Lewis, S. W., Kilcommons, A., Green, J., et al. (2004). Cognitive therapy for the prevention of psychosis in people at ultra-high risk: randomised controlled trial. *British Journal of Psychiatry*, 185, 291–297.
31. Falloon, I. R. (1992). Early intervention for first episodes of schizophrenia: A preliminary exploration. *Psychiatry*, 55(1), 4–15.
32. Chapman, L. J., & Chapman, J. P. (1987). The search for symptoms predictive of schizophrenia. *Schizophrenia Bulletin*, 13(3), 497–503.
33. Chapman, L. J., Chapman, J. P., Kwapil, T. R., Eckblad, M., & Zinser, M. C. (1994). Putatively psychosis-prone subjects 10 years later. *Journal of Abnormal Psychology*, 103(2), 171–183.
34. Huber, G., Gross, G., Schuttler, R., & Linz, M. (1980). Longitudinal studies of schizophrenic patients. *Schizophrenia Bulletin*, 6(4), 592–605.
35. Klosterkotter, J., Hellmich, M., Steinmeyer, E. M., & Schultze-Lutter, F. (2001). Diagnosing schizophrenia in the initial prodromal phase. *Archives of General Psychiatry*, 58(2), 158–164.
36. Yung, A. R., & McGorry, P. D. (1996). The prodromal phase of first-episode psychosis: Past and current conceptualizations. *Schizophrenia Bulletin*, 22(2), 353–370.
37. Yung, A. R., McGorry, P. D., McFarlane, C. A., Jackson, H. J., Patton, G. C., & Rakkar, A. (1996). Monitoring and care of young people at incipient risk of psychosis. *Schizophrenia Bulletin*, 22(2), 283–303.
38. Yung, A. R., Phillips, L. J., Yuen, H. P., Francey, S. M., McFarlane, C. A., Hallgren, M., et al. (2003). Psychosis prediction: Twelve-month follow-up of a high-risk ("prodromal") group. *Schizophrenia Research*, 60(1), 21–32.
39. Jones, P., & van Os, J. (1997). Predicting schizophrenia in teenagers: Pessimistic results from the British 1946 birth cohort. Paper presented at the Sixth International Conference on Schizophrenia Research. Colorado Springs.
40. Davidson, M., Reichenberg, A., Rabinowitz, J., Weiser, M., Kaplan, Z., & Mark, M. (1999). Behavioral and intellectual markers for schizophrenia in apparently healthy male adolescents. *American Journal of Psychiatry*, 156(9), 1328–1335.

41. Jones, P., & Croudace, T. (2001). Predicting schizophrenia from teachers' reports of behavior. In T. Miller et al. (Eds.), *Early Intervention in Psychotic Disorders* (pp. 1–28). Dordrecht: Kluwer Academic Publishing.
42. Varsamis, J., & Adamson, J. D. (1971). Early schizophrenia. *Canadian Psychiatric Association Journal*, 16(6), 487–497.
43. Miller, T. J., McGlashan, T. H., Woods, S. W., Stein, K., Driesen, N., Corcoran, C. M., et al. (1999). Symptom assessment in schizophrenic prodromal states. *Psychiatric Quarterly*, 70(4), 273–287.
44. McGlashan, T., Miller, T., Woods, S. W., Hoffman, R., & Davidson, L. (2001). Instrument for the assessment of prodromal symptoms and states. In T. Miller et al. (Eds.), *Early Intervention in Psychotic Disorders* (pp. 135–139). Netherlands: Kluwer Academic Publishers.
45. Overall, J.E., & Gorham, D.R. (1962). The Brief Psychiatric Rating Scale. *Psychology Report*, 10, 799–812.
46. Kay, S. R., Fiszbein, A., & Opler, L. A. (1987). The positive and negative syndrome scale (PANSS) for schizophrenia. *Schizophrenia Bulletin*, 13(2), 261–276.
47. Andreasen, N. C., Flaum, M., & Arndt, S. (1992). The Comprehensive Assessment of Symptoms and History (CASH): An instrument for assessing diagnosis and psychopathology. *Archives of General Psychiatry*, 49(8), 615–623.
48. American Psychiatric Association. (1994). *Diagnostic and Statistical Manual of Mental Disorders, Fourth Edition (DSM-IV)*. Washington, D.C.: American Psychiatric Association.
49. Yung, A. R. (2006). Identification of the population. In J. Addington (Ed.), *Working with People at High Risk of Developing Psychosis* (pp. 7–23). Hoboken, NJ: John Wiley & Sons.
50. Miller, T.J., McGlashan, T.H., Rosen, J.L., Cadenhead, K., Ventura, J., et al. (2003). Prodromal assessment with the Structured Interview for Prodromal Syndromes and the Scale of Prodromal Symptoms: Predictive validity, interrater reliability, and training to reliability. *Schizophrenia Bulletin*, 29(4), 703–715.
51. Cannon, T. D., Cadenhead, K., Cornblatt, B., Woods, S. W., Addington, J., Walker, E., et al. (2008). Prediction of psychosis in youth at high clinical risk: A multisite longitudinal study in North America. *Archives of General Psychiatry*, 65(1), 28–37.
52. Hawkins, K. A., McGlashan, T. H., Quinlan, D., Miller, T. J., Perkins, D. O., Zipursky, R. B., et al. (2004). Factorial structure of the scale of prodromal symptoms. *Schizophrenia Research* 68(2–3):339–347.
53. Hall, R. C. (1995). Global assessment of functioning. A modified scale. *Psychosomatics*, 36(3), 267–275.
54. Woods, S. W., Miller, T., & McGlashan, T. (2001). The "prodromal patient": Both symptomatic and at-risk. *CNS Spectrums*, 6(3), 223–232.
55. Guy, W. (1976). *ECDEU Assessment Manual for Psychopharmacology, rev. ed.* Bethesda: Department of Health, Education, and Welfare.
56. Montgomery, S. A., & Asberg, M. (1979). A new depression scale designed to be sensitive to change. *British Journal of Psychiatry*, 134, 382–389.

57. Young, R. C., Biggs, J. T., Ziegler, V. E., & Meyer, D. A. (1978). A rating scale for mania: Reliability, validity, and sensitivity. *British Journal of Psychiatry*, 133, 429–435.
58. Baker, F., & Intagliata, J. (1982). Quality of life in the evaluation of community support systems. *Evaluation & Program Planning*, 5(1), 69–79.
59. Cannon-Spoor, H. E., Potkin, S. G., & Wyatt, R. J. (1982). Measurement of premorbid adjustment in chronic schizophrenia. *Schizophrenia Bulletin*, 8(3), 470–484.
60. Zimmerman, M., Coryell, W., Pfohl, B., & Stangl, D. (1988). The reliability of the family history method for psychiatric diagnoses. *Archives of General Psychiatry*, 45(4), 320–322.
61. Lencz, T., Smith, C. W., Auther, A., Correll, C. U., & Cornblatt, B. (2004). Nonspecific and attenuated negative symptoms in patients at clinical high-risk for schizophrenia. *Schizophrenia Research*, 68(1), 37–48.
62. Meyer, S. E., Bearden, C. E., Lux, S. R., Gordon, J. L., Johnson, J. K., O'Brien, M. P., et al. (2005). The psychosis prodrome in adolescent patients viewed through the lens of DSM-IV. *Journal of Child & Adolescent Psychopharmacology*, 15(3), 434–451.
63. McGlashan, T. H., Zipursky, R. B., Perkins, D., Addington, J., Miller, T. J., Woods, S. W., et al. (2003). The PRIME North America randomized double-blind clinical trial of olanzapine versus placebo in patients at risk of being prodromally symptomatic for psychosis. I. Study rationale and design. *Schizophrenia Research*, 61(1), 7–18.
64. Woods, S. W., Breier, A., Zipursky, R. B., Perkins, D. O., Addington, J., Miller, T. J., et al. (2003). Randomized trial of olanzapine versus placebo in the symptomatic acute treatment of the schizophrenic prodrome. [erratum appears in *Biol Psychiatry*. 2003 Aug 15;54(4):497]. *Biological Psychiatry*, 54(4), 453–464.
65. Rosen, J. L., Miller, T. J., D'Andrea, J. T., McGlashan, T. H., & Woods, S. W. (2006). Comorbid diagnoses in patients meeting criteria for the schizophrenia prodrome. *Schizophrenia Research*, 85(1–3), 124–131.
66. First, M. B., Spitzer, R. L., Gibbon, M., & Williams, J. B. W. *Structured Clinical Interview for DSMIV Axis I Disorders—Patient Edition (SCID-I/P, Version 2.0)*. Psychiatric Institute, New York: Biometric Research Department.
67. Zanarini, M. C., Frankenburg, F. R., Chauncey, D. L., & Gunderson, J. G. (1987). The diagnostic Interview for Personality Disorders: Interrater and test-retest reliability. *Comprehensive Psychiatry*, 28(6), 467–480.
68. McGlashan, T.H. (2003). Commentary: Progress, issues, and implications of prodromal research: An inside view. *Schizophrenia Bulletin*, 29, 851–858.
69. Kaufman, J., Birmaher, B., Brent, D. Rao, U., Flynn, C., Moreci, P., et al. (1997). Schedule for Affective Disorders and Schizophrenia for School-Age Children-Present and Lifetime Version (K-SADS-PL): Initial reliability and validity data. *Journal of the American Academy of Child & Adolescent Psychiatry*, 36, 980–988.

Appendix A

Risk Syndrome Phone Screen

Screen number: ___________

Screen date: ___________ Eligible for Evaluation: Yes No

Screener: ___________ Date of Evaluation: ___________

PRIME CLINIC PHONE SCREEN

Patient Information:

Name: ____

Age: ___________ **D.O.B.:** ___________ **Male** **Female**

Telephone (home): _____________ **Telephone (other):**_____________

Address:____

Has verbal consent been given to permanently retain PHI?
☐ **Yes** ☐ **No**

Daytime activity (e.g. work/school):________________________

Referrer Information:

Name: ____________________ **Relationship to Patient:** ________________

Organization: ____

Tel. 1: ________________ **Tel. 2:** ________________ **Tel. 3:** ______________

Address: ____

____

If referrer is a health provider; is referrer willing to be included in the community provider directory? ☐ **Yes** ☐ **No**

Describe area(s) of expertise (e.g. age group, diagnosis):

How did you learn about the PRIME Clinic?

____

Clinical Information:

1. **What prompted you to call PRIME?** (Obtain an account of clinical changes.) Query the onset and duration of symptoms. If no relevant symptoms are presented, record information the caller can report. Inquire about:
   - Changes in thinking (odd ideas, grandiosity, suspiciousness, difficulty concentrating)
   - Changes in perception (auditory/visual/tactile/olfactory abnormalities)
   - Changes in speech (disorganized communication, tangential speech)
   - Changes in perception (of self, others, or the world in general)
   - Vegetative symptoms (sleep problems, changes in appetite, social isolation)
   - Emotional changes (depression, mood swings, irritability, flat affect)
   - Family history of mental illness
   - Dramatic reduction of overall functioning

____

____

____

____

____

2. **Have these symptoms and/or changes been related to any medication or drug use?**

   Yes No

3. **Does the patient have a past or current medical history of a clinically significant central nervous system disorder (i.e., seizure disorder) that could explain prodromal symptoms?**

   Yes No

   Describe:

4. **Psychiatric History/History of Impaired Intellectual Functioning (i.e., IQ<65)?**

   Yes No

   Describe (e.g., diagnoses, provider, treatment):

5. **Medication History?**

   Yes No

   Antipsychotic medication in the past week?

   Yes No

Antipsychotic medication received for greater than 16 weeks in patient's lifetime?

Yes No

____

____

____

List All Medications Reported:

Medication	Current/Past	Dosage	Duration of use	Reason(s) prescribed

6. **Family History of Mental Illness?**

Yes No

Describe:

____

____

____

Summary Worksheet:

1. **Is the patient between the ages of 12 and 35?**

Yes No

2. **Symptom Checklist:**

Symptom	Yes	No	Symptom Description/Onset/Duration
Changes in perception			(e.g., auditory/visual/tactile/olfactory abnormalities)
Changes in speech, thinking			(e.g., odd ideas, suspiciousness, difficulty concentrating, tangential speech, grandiosity)
Changes in functioning			(e.g., work/academic difficulties, social isolation)

Changes in emotions			(e.g., flat affect, depression, anxiety, mood swings, irritability)
Vegetative symptoms			(e.g., sleep difficulties, changes in appetite, somatic complaints)
Other reported changes			

1. **Using the Symptom Checklist, is the patient reporting any recent changes?**

   Yes No

2. **Does the patient have a history of impaired intellectual functioning (i.e., IQ<65)?**

   Yes No

3. **Does the patient have a nervous system disorder that could explain prodromal symptoms?**

   Yes No

4. **Has the patient ever been diagnosed with/treated for a psychotic disorder?**

   Yes No

If the answer to #1 is yes, and the rest are no, the patient is eligible to be evaluated.

Appendix B

SIPS/SOPS 5.0

STRUCTURED INTERVIEW FOR PSYCHOSIS-RISK SYNDROMES

ENGLISH LANGUAGE

Thomas H. McGlashan, MD
Barbara C. Walsh, PhD
Scott W. Woods, MD

PRIME Research Clinic Yale School of Medicine
New Haven, Connecticut USA

CONTRIBUTORS

Jean Addington, PhD, Kristin Cadenhead, MD, Tyrone Cannon, PhD, Barbara Cornblatt, PhD, Larry Davidson, PhD, Robert Heinssen, PhD, Ralph Hoffman, MD, TK Larsen, MD, Tandy Miller, PhD, Diane Perkins, MD, Larry Seidman, PhD, Joanna Rosen, PsyD, Ming Tsuang, MD, PhD, Elaine Walker, PhD

January 1, 2010
Version 5.0

Table of Contents

STRUCTURED INTERVIEW FOR PSYCHOSIS-RISK SYNDROMES

Overview:

The aims of the interview are to:

I Rule out past and/or current psychosis
II Rule in one or more of the three types of psychosis-risk syndromes
III Rate the current severity of the psychosis-risk symptoms

I. Rule Out a Past and/or Current Psychotic Syndrome

A past psychosis should be ruled out using information obtained through either the initial screen or the Overview (pp. 187–188) and evaluated using the Presence of Psychotic Symptoms criteria (POPS).

Current psychosis is defined by the presence of Positive Symptoms. Ruling out a current psychosis requires the questioning of and rating on the five Positive Symptom items outlined in the measure: Unusual Thought Content/Delusions, Suspiciousness, Grandiosity, Perceptual Abnormalities/Hallucinations, and Disorganized Speech.

PRESENCE OF PSYCHOTIC SYMPTOMS CRITERIA (POPS)

Current psychosis is defined as follows:
Both **(A)** and **(B)** are required.

(A) Positive Symptoms are present at a psychotic level of intensity (*Rated at level "6"*):

- Unusual thought content, suspiciousness/persecution, or grandiosity with delusional conviction

AND/OR

- Perceptual abnormality of hallucinatory intensity

AND/OR

- Speech that is incoherent or unintelligible

(B) Any **(A)** criterion symptom at sufficient frequency and duration or urgency:

- At least one symptom from **(A)** has occurred over a period of one month for at least one hour per day at a minimum average frequency of four days per week

OR

- Symptom that is seriously disorganizing or dangerous

Positive Symptoms are rated on scales P1–P5 of the Scale of Psychosis-risk Symptoms (SOPS). A score of "1" to "5" on one or more of scales P1–P5 indicates a Positive Symptom that is at a non-psychotic level of intensity. A score of "6" on one or more of scales P1–P5 indicates that a Positive Symptom is at a *"Severe and Psychotic"* level of intensity, and thus the **(A)** criteria is met.

The presence of a current psychosis, however, depends also upon the frequency or urgency of the **(A)** criterion symptom(s). If a Positive Symptom also satisfies the **(B)** criterion, a current psychosis is defined.

II. Rule in One or More of the Three Types of Psychosis-Risk Syndromes

(Criteria Summaries on p. 235).

PLEASE NOTE THAT THE THREE PSYCHOSIS-RISK STATES ARE NOT MUTUALLY EXCLUSIVE. PATIENTS CAN MEET CRITERIA FOR ONE OR MORE SYNDROME TYPES.

Patients not meeting criteria for a past or current psychosis are evaluated on the Criteria of Psychosis-risk Syndromes (COPS) for the presence of one or more of the three psychosis-risk syndromes: Brief Intermittent Psychotic Syndrome, Attenuated Positive Symptom Syndrome, and Genetic Risk and Deterioration Syndrome.

Criteria of Psychosis-risk Syndromes:

1. **Brief Intermittent Psychotic Syndrome (BIPS)**
   The Brief Intermittent Psychotic Syndrome is defined by frankly psychotic symptoms that are recent and very brief. To meet criteria for BIPS, a psychotic intensity symptom (SOPS score = 6) must have begun in the past three months and must be present at least several minutes a day at a frequency of at least once per month. Even if these Positive Symptoms are present at a psychotic level of intensity (SOPS score = 6), a current psychotic syndrome can be ruled out if the POPS **(B)** criteria for sufficient frequency and duration or urgency are not met.
2. **Attenuated Positive Symptom Syndrome (APSS)**
   The Attenuated Positive Symptom Syndrome is defined by the presence of recent attenuated positive symptoms of sufficient severity and frequency. To meet criteria for an attenuated symptom, a patient must receive a rating of level "3", "4", or "5" on scales P1–P5 of the SOPS. A rating in this range indicates a symptom severity that is at a psychosis-risk level of intensity.

   Also, the symptom must either have begun in the past year or must currently rate at least one scale point higher than it would if rated 12 months ago. Second, the symptom must occur at the current intensity level at an average frequency of at least once per week in the past month.
3. **Genetic Risk and Deterioration Syndrome (GRDS)**
   The Genetic Risk and Deterioration Syndrome is defined by a combined genetic risk for a schizophrenic spectrum disorder and recent functional

deterioration. The genetic risk criterion can be met if the patient has a first degree relative with any affective or nonaffective psychotic disorder and/or the patient meets criteria for DSM-IV Schizotypal Personality Disorder criteria.

Functional deterioration is operationally defined as a 30% or greater drop in the GAF score during the last month compared to the patient's highest GAF score in the prior 12 months.

III. Rate the Current Severity of the Psychosis-risk Symptoms

Patients meeting criteria for one or more psychosis-risk syndromes are further evaluated using the SOPS rating scales for Negative Symptoms, Disorganization Symptoms, and General Symptoms. While this additional information will not contribute to the diagnosis of a psychosis-risk syndrome, it will provide both a descriptive and quantitative estimate of the diversity and severity of psychosis-risk symptoms. Some investigators may wish to obtain a full SOPS with all patients.

SCALE OF PSYCHOSIS-RISK SYMPTOMS (SOPS)

Instructions for Using the Rating Scales:

The SOPS describes and rates psychosis-risk and other symptoms that have occurred in the past month (or since the last rating if more recently).

The SOPS is organized in four primary sections: **(P.) Positive Symptoms, (N.) Negative Symptoms, (D.) Disorganization Symptoms, (G.) General Symptoms.** The SOPS final ratings are recorded on a summary sheet located at the end of the SIPS.

INQUIRY

Within each section of the SOPS, a series of questions are listed with space provided for recording responses ("N" = No; "NI"= No Information; "Y" = Yes). **All boldface inquiries should be asked.** Questions that are not printed in boldface are optional and can be included for clarification or elaboration of positive responses.

QUALIFIERS

Following each set of questions, a series of qualifiers is listed. Each question that elicits a positive (i.e., "Y") response should be followed by these qualifiers in order to obtain more detailed information. The qualifier box is listed below:

QUALIFIERS: For all "Y" responses, record:

- Description-Onset-Duration-Frequency
- Degree of Distress: What is this experience like for you? Does it bother you?
- Degree of interference with life: Do you ever act on this experience? Does having the experience ever cause you to do anything differently?
- Degree of Conviction/Meaning: How do you account for this experience? Do you ever feel that it could just be in your head? Do you think this is real?

SCALES

Two different severity scales are used for measuring indicated symptoms. Positive Symptoms are rated on one severity scale while Negative, Disorganization, and General Symptoms are rated using a second severity scale.

Anchors in each scale are intended to provide guidelines and examples of signs for every symptom observed. It is not necessary to meet every criterion in any one anchor to assign a particular rating. When patients meet some criteria within one anchor and some criteria within an adjacent anchor such that a clear anchor cannot be chosen, rate to the extreme. Basis for ratings includes both interviewer observations and patient reports. Third-party reports alone do not qualify.

Both scales are listed below.

Positive Symptoms Scale:
Positive Symptoms are rated on a SOPS scale that ranges from 0 (Absent) to 6 (Severe and Psychotic):

Positive Symptom SOPS

0	1	2	3	4	5	6
Absent	Questionably Present	Mild	Moderate	Moderately Severe	Severe but Not Psychotic	Severe and Psychotic

Negative/Disorganized/General Symptoms Scale:

Negative/Disorganized/General Symptom Symptoms are rated on a SOPS scale that ranges from 0 (Absent) to 6 (Extreme):

Negative/Disorganized/General Symptom SOPS

0	1	2	3	4	5	6
Absent	Questionably Present	Mild	Moderate	Moderately Severe	Severe	Extreme

RATING RATIONALE

Each severity scale is followed by a "**Rating based on:**" section. After a rating is assigned, provide a brief description of the symptom(s) and the rationale for assigning the specific rating.

SYMPTOM ONSET, WORSENING, AND FREQUENCY

Following each **Rating based on:** section, a four-part rating box is shown.

For Positive symptoms rated at a level 3 or higher, under Symptom Onset record the date when the earliest symptom first occurred in the 3–6 range.

Under Symptom Worsening, record the most recent date when the symptom increased in severity by one point. Under Symptom Frequency, check the boxes that map onto the COPS criteria. For Negative, Disorganization, and General Symptoms, an abbreviated symptom onset box is listed.

Under Better Explained, also rate for positive symptoms whether the symptom is better explained by an Axis I or Axis II disorder. There are two tests.

The first test is temporal sequence. If the positive symptoms were present before onset of the co-occurring disorder or persist when the co-occurring diagnosis is in remission, rate NOT better explained. If the co-occurring diagnosis has been present continuously during the period of positive symptoms, the second test is applied.

The second test is whether the positive symptoms are more characteristic of a psychosis-risk syndrome or of the co-occurring disorder. When the positive symptoms are more characteristic of the other disorder, the symptoms are considered better explained by the other disorder. For example: feelings of impending death during a panic attack are better explained by panic disorder than by a psychosis risk-syndrome, feelings of personal worthlessness in a depressed patient are better explained by depression than by a psychosis-risk syndrome, feelings of personal superiority in a patient with frank mania is better explained by the mania, and feelings of personal disintegration precipitated by stress and relieved by wrist-cutting in a borderline patient is better explained by the personality disorder. The sole exception is for schizotypal personality disorder: Positive symptoms that are worsening are always rated as NOT better explained by the disorder.

In cases of ambiguity, tend toward rating NOT better explained. For example, momentary illusions of "black shadows" with vague persecutory intent in a patient with comorbid depression is rated as NOT better explained, because such illusions are more characteristic of a risk syndrome than depression, despite the possibility that the "black" quality could relate to depressive themes.

For Symptoms Rated at Level 3 or Higher			
Symptom Onset	**Symptom Worsening**	**Symptom Frequency**	**Better Explained**
Record date when a positive symptom first reached at least a 3: ☐ "Ever since I can recall" ☐ Date of onset ___/___Month/Year	Record most recent date when a positive symptom currently rated 3-6 experienced an increase by at least one rating point: Date of worsening ___/___Month/Year	Check all that apply: ☐ ≥ 1h/d, ≥ 4d/wk ☐ ≥ several minutes/d, ≥ 1x/mo ☐ ≥ 1x/wk ☐ none of above	Symptoms are better explained by another Axis I or II disorder. Check one: ☐ Likely ☐ Not likely

Overview:

The purpose of the overview is to obtain information about what has brought the person to the interview, recent functioning, and educational, developmental, occupational, and social history.

The overview should include:

- Any behaviors and symptoms obtained from the phone screen or prescreen (if applicable).
- Occupational or academic functioning history, including any recent changes. Include participation in special education programs.
- Developmental history
- Social history and any recent changes
- Trauma history
- History of substance use

Now I'd like to ask you some more general questions. How have things been going for you recently?

Overview (cont'd):

FAMILY HISTORY OF MENTAL ILLNESS

1. Who are your first-degree relatives (i.e., parent, full sibling, half-child)?

Relationship	Age	Name	History of mental illness? (Y/N)

2. For those first-degree relatives who have a history of mental illness:

Name of relative	Name of problem	Symptoms	Duration	Treatment history

3. Does the patient have any first-degree relatives with a psychotic disorder (Schizophrenia, Schizophreniform Disorder, Brief Psychosis, Delusional Disorder, Psychotic Disorder NOS, Schizoaffective Disorder, Psychotic Mania, Psychotic Depression)? Yes___ No___

P. POSITIVE SYMPTOMS

P. 1. UNUSUAL THOUGHT CONTENT/DELUSIONAL IDEAS

The following questions are organized in sections and probe for both psychotic, delusional thinking and for non-psychotic, unusual thought content.

These experiences are rated on the SOPS P1 Scale at the end of the queries.

Y=YES N=NO NI=NO INFORMATION

PERPLEXITY AND DELUSIONAL MOOD

Inquiry:

1. **Have you had the feeling that something odd is going on or that something is wrong that you can't explain?**	**N**	**NI**	**Y**	**(Record Qualifiers)**
2. **Have you ever been confused at times whether something you have experienced is real or imaginary?**	**N**	**NI**	**Y**	**(Record Qualifiers)**
3. **Do familiar people or surroundings ever seem strange?** Confusing? Unreal? Not a part of the living world? Alien? Inhuman? Evil?	**N**	**NI**	**Y**	**(Record Qualifiers)**
4. **Does your experience of time seem to have changed? Unnaturally faster, unnaturally slower?**	**N**	**NI**	**Y**	**(Record Qualifiers)**
5. **Do you ever seem to live through events exactly as you have experienced them before?**	**N**	**NI**	**Y**	**(Record Qualifiers)**

QUALIFIERS: For all "Y" responses, record:

- Description-Onset-Duration-Frequency
- Degree of Distress: What is this experience like for you? (Does it bother you?)
- Degree of interference with life: Do you ever act on this experience? Does having the experience ever cause you to do anything differently?
- Degree of Conviction/Meaning: How do you account for this experience? Do you ever feel that it could just be in your head? Do you think this is real?

FIRST-RANK SYMPTOMS

Inquiry:

1. **Have you felt that you are not in control of your own ideas or thoughts?**	N	NI	Y	(Record Qualifiers)
2. **Do you ever feel as if somehow thoughts are put into your head or taken away from you?** Do you ever feel that some person or force may be controlling or interfering with your thinking?	N	NI	Y	(Record Qualifiers)
3. **Do you ever feel as if your thoughts are being said out loud so that other people can hear them?**	N	NI	Y	(Record Qualifiers)
4. **Do you ever think that people might be able to read your mind?**	N	NI	Y	(Record Qualifiers)
5. **Do you ever think that you can read other people's minds?**	N	NI	Y	(Record Qualifiers)
6. **Do you ever feel the radio or TV is communicating directly to you?**	N	NI	Y	(Record Qualifiers)

QUALIFIERS: For all "Y" responses, record:

- Description-Onset-Duration-Frequency
- Degree of Distress: What is this experience like for you? (Does it bother you?)
- Degree of interference with life: Do you ever act on this experience? Does having the experience ever cause you to do anything differently?
- Degree of Conviction/Meaning: How do you account for this experience? Do you ever feel that it could just be in your head? Do you think this is real?

OVERVALUED BELIEFS

Inquiry:

1. **Do you have strong feelings or beliefs that are very important to you, about such things as religion, philosophy, or politics?**	**N**	**NI**	**Y**	**(Record Qualifiers)**
2. **Do you daydream a lot or find yourself preoccupied with stories, fantasies, or ideas?** Do you ever feel confused about whether something is your imagination or real?	**N**	**NI**	**Y**	**(Record Qualifiers)**
3. **Do you know what it means to be superstitious? Are you superstitious? Does it affect your behavior?**	**N**	**NI**	**Y**	**(Record Qualifiers)**
4. **Do other people tell you that your ideas or beliefs are unusual or bizarre?** **If so, what are these ideas or beliefs?**	**N**	**NI**	**Y**	**(Record Qualifiers)**
5. **Do you ever feel you can predict the future?**	**N**	**NI**	**Y**	**(Record Qualifiers)**

QUALIFIERS: For all "Y" responses, record:

- Description-Onset-Duration-Frequency
- Degree of Distress: What is this experience like for you? (Does it bother you?)
- Degree of interference with life: Do you ever act on this experience? Does having the experience ever cause you to do anything differently?
- Degree of Conviction/Meaning: How do you account for this experience? Do you ever feel that it could just be in your head? Do you think this is real?

____

____

____

____

____

OTHER UNUSUAL THOUGHTS/DELUSIONAL IDEAS

Inquiry:

1. **Somatic Ideas: Do you ever worry that something might be wrong with your body or your health?**	**N**	**NI**	**Y**	**(Record Qualifiers)**
2. **Nihilistic Ideas: Have you ever felt that you might not actually exist?** Do you ever think that the world might not exist?	**N**	**NI**	**Y**	**(Record Qualifiers)**
3. **Ideas of Guilt: Do you ever find yourself thinking a lot about how to be good or begin to believe that you deserve to be punished in some way?**	**N**	**NI**	**Y**	**(Record Qualifiers)**

____
____
____
____
____
____
____
____

NON-PERSECUTORY IDEAS OF REFERENCE

Inquiry:

1. **Have you felt that things happening around you have a special meaning for just you?**	**N**	**NI**	**Y**	**(Record Qualifiers)**
2. **Have you had the sense that you are often the center of people's attention?** Do you feel they have hostile or negative intentions?	**N**	**NI**	**Y**	**(Record Qualifiers)**

QUALIFIERS: For all "Y" responses, record:

- Description-Onset-Duration-Frequency
- Degree of Distress: What is this experience like for you? (Does it bother you?)
- Degree of interference with life: Do you ever act on this experience? Does having the experience ever cause you to do anything differently?
- Degree of Conviction/Meaning: How do you account for this experience? Do you ever feel that it could just be in your head? Do you think this is real?

P. 1. DESCRIPTION: UNUSUAL THOUGHT CONTENT/ DELUSIONAL IDEAS

a. Perplexity and delusional mood. Mind tricks, such as the sense that something odd is going on or puzzlement and confusion about what is real or imaginary. The familiar feels strange, confusing, ominous, threatening, or has special meaning. Sense that self, others, the world have changed. Changes in perception of time. Déjà vu experience.
b. Non-persecutory ideas of reference.
c. First-rank phenomenology. Mental events such as thought insertion/ interference/withdrawal/broadcasting/telepathy/external control/radio and TV messages.
d. Overvalued beliefs. Preoccupation with unusually valued ideas (religion, meditation, philosophy, existential themes). Magical thinking that influences behavior and is inconsistent with subculture norms (e.g., being superstitious, belief in clairvoyance, uncommon religious beliefs).
e. Unusual ideas about the body, guilt, nihilism, jealousy, and religion. Delusions may be present but are not well organized and not tenaciously held.

Anchors in each scale are intended to provide guidelines and examples of signs for every symptom observed. It is not necessary to meet every criterion in any one anchor to assign a particular rating. Basis for ratings includes both interviewer observations and patient reports.

UNUSUAL THOUGHT CONTENT/DELUSIONAL IDEAS **Severity Scale (circle one)**

0 Absent	1 Questionably Present	2 Mild	3 Moderate	4 Moderately Severe	5 Severe but Not Psychotic	6 Severe and Psychotic
	"Mind tricks" that are puzzling. Sense that something is different.	Overly interested in fantasy life. Unusually valued ideas/ beliefs. Some superstitions beyond what might be expected by the average person but within cultural norms.	Unanticipated mental events that are puzzling, unwilled, but not easily ignored. Experiences seem meaningful because they recur and will not go away. Functions mostly as usual.	Sense that ideas/ experiences/ beliefs may be coming from outside oneself or that they may be real, but doubt remains intact. Distracting, bothersome. May affect functioning.	Experiences familiar, anticipated. Doubt can be induced by contrary evidence and others' opinions. Distressingly real. Affects daily functioning.	Delusional conviction (with no doubt) at least intermittently. Interferes persistently with thinking, feeling, social relations, and/or behavior.

Rating based on: ____

____

____

____

For Symptoms Rated at Level 3 or Higher			
Symptom Onset	**Symptom Worsening**	**Symptom Frequency**	**Better Explained**
Record date when a positive symptom first reached at least a 3: ☐ "Ever since I can recall" ☐ Date of onset ___/___Month/Year	Record most recent date when a positive symptom currently rated 3-6 experienced an increase by at least one rating point Date of worsening ___/___Month/ Year	Check all that apply: ☐ ≥ 1h/d, ≥ 4d/wk ☐ ≥ several minutes/d, ≥1x/mo ☐ ≥ 1x/wk ☐ none of above	Symptoms are better explained by another Axis I or II disorder. Check one: ☐ Likely ☐ Not likely

P. 2. SUSPICIOUSNESS/PERSECUTORY IDEAS

The following questions probe for paranoid ideas of reference, paranoid thinking, or suspiciousness. They are rated on the SOPS P2 Scale at the end of the queries.

SUSPICIOUSNESS/PERSECUTORY IDEAS

Inquiry:

1. **Do you ever feel that people around you are thinking about you in a negative way?** Have you ever found out later that this was not true or that your suspicions were unfounded?	N	NI	Y	(Record Qualifiers)
2. **Have you ever found yourself feeling mistrustful or suspicious of other people?**	N	NI	Y	(Record Qualifiers)
3. **Do you ever feel that you have to pay close attention to what's going on around you in order to feel safe?**	N	NI	Y	(Record Qualifiers)
4. **Do you ever feel like you are being singled out or watched?**	N	NI	Y	(Record Qualifiers)
5. **Do you ever feel people might be intending to harm you?** Do you have a sense of who that might be?	N	NI	Y	(Record Qualifiers)

QUALIFIERS: For all "Y" responses, record:

- Description-Onset-Duration-Frequency
- Degree of Distress: What is this experience like for you? (Does it bother you?)
- Degree of interference with life: Do you ever act on this experience? Does having the experience ever cause you to do anything differently?
- Degree of Conviction/Meaning: How do you account for this experience? Do you ever feel that it could just be in your head? Do you think this is real?

P.2. DESCRIPTION: SUSPICIOUSNESS/PERSECUTORY IDEAS

a. Persecutory ideas of reference.
b. Suspiciousness or paranoid thinking.
c. Presents a guarded or even openly distrustful attitude that may reflect delusional conviction and intrude on the interview and/or behavior.

Anchors in each scale are intended to provide guidelines and examples of signs for every symptom observed. It is not necessary to meet every criterion in any one anchor to assign a particular rating. Basis for ratings includes both interviewer observations and patient reports.

SUSPICIOUSNESS/PERSECUTORY IDEAS **Severity Scale (circle one)**

0 Absent	1 Questionably Present	2 Mild	3 Moderate	4 Moderately Severe	5 Severe but Not Psychotic	6 Severe and Psychotic
	Wariness.	Concerns about safety. Hypervigilance without clear source of danger.	Concerns that people are untrustworthy and/or may harbor ill will. Sense of unease and need for vigilance (often unfocused). Mistrustful. Recurrent (yet unfounded) sense that people might be thinking or saying negative things about person.	Thoughts of being the object of negative attention. Sense that people may wish harm. Self-generated skepticism present. Preoccupying, distressing. May affect daily functioning. May appear defensive in response to questioning.	Beliefs about danger from hostile intentions of others. Skepticism and perspective can prevail with non-confirming evidence or other's opinion. Anxious, unsettled. Daily functioning affected. Guarded presentation may diminish information gathered in the interview.	Delusional paranoid conviction (no doubt) at least intermittently. Frightened, avoidant, watchful. Interferes persistently with thinking, feeling, social relations, and/or behavior.

Rating based on:____

____

____

____

____

____

____

For Symptoms Rated at Level 3 or Higher			
Symptom Onset	**Symptom Worsening**	**Symptom Frequency**	**Better Explained**
Record date when a positive symptom first reached at least a 3: ☐ "Ever since I can recall" ☐ Date of onset ___/___Month/Year	Record most recent date when a positive symptom currently rated 3-6 experienced an increase by at least one rating point Date of worsening ___/___Month/Year	Check all that apply: ☐ ≥ 1h/d, ≥ 4d/wk ☐ ≥ several minutes/d, ≥x/mo ☐ ≥ 1x/wk ☐ none of above	Symptoms are better explained by another Axis I or II disorder Check one: ☐ Likely ☐ Not likely

P. 3. GRANDIOSE IDEAS

The following questions probe for psychotic grandiosity, non-psychotic grandiosity, and inflated self-esteem. They are rated on the SOPS P3 Scale at the end of the queries.

GRANDIOSE IDEAS

Inquiry:

1. **Do you feel you have special gifts or talents?** Do you feel as if you are unusually gifted in any particular area? Do you talk about your gifts with other people?	N	NI	Y	**(Record Qualifiers)**
2. **Have you ever behaved without regard to painful consequences? For example, do you ever go on excessive spending sprees that you can't afford?**	N	NI	Y	**(Record Qualifiers)**
3. **Do people ever tell you that your plans or goals are unrealistic? What are these plans? How do you imagine accomplishing them?**	N	NI	Y	**(Record Qualifiers)**
4. **Do you ever think of yourself as a famous or particularly important person?**	N	NI	Y	**(Record Qualifiers)**
5. **Do you ever feel that you have been chosen by God for a special role?** Do you ever feel as if you can save others?	N	NI	Y	**(Record Qualifiers)**

QUALIFIERS: For all "Y" responses, record:

- Description-Onset-Duration-Frequency
- Degree of Distress: What is this experience like for you? (Does it bother you?)
- Degree of interference with life: Do you ever act on this experience? Does having the experience ever cause you to do anything differently?
- Degree of Conviction/Meaning: How do you account for this experience? Do you ever feel that it could just be in your head? Do you think this is real?

P.3. DESCRIPTION: GRANDIOSE IDEAS

a. Exaggerated self-opinion and unrealistic sense of superiority.
b. Some expansiveness or boastfulness.
c. Occasional clear-cut grandiose delusions that can influence behavior.

Anchors in each scale are intended to provide guidelines and examples of signs for every symptom observed. It is not necessary to meet every criterion in any one anchor to assign a particular rating. Basis for ratings includes both interviewer observations and patient reports.

GRANDIOSE IDEAS **Severity Scale (circle one)**

0 Absent	1 Questionably Present	2 Mild	3 Moderate	4 Moderately Severe	5 Severe but Not Psychotic	6 Severe and Psychotic
	Private thoughts of being better than others.	Mostly private thoughts of being talented, understanding, or gifted.	Notions of being unusually gifted, powerful or special and have exaggerated expectations. May be expansive but can redirect to the everyday on own.	Beliefs of talent, influence, and abilities. Unrealistic goals that may affect plans and functioning, but responsive to other's concerns and limits.	Compelling beliefs of superior intellect, attractiveness, power, or fame. Skepticism and modesty can only be elicited by the efforts of others. Affects functioning.	Delusions of grandiosity with conviction (no doubt) at least intermittently Interferes persistently with thinking, feeling, social relations, or behavior.

Rating based on:____

____
____
____
____
____
____
____

For Symptoms Rated at Level 3 or Higher			
Symptom Onset	**Symptom Worsening**	**Symptom Frequency**	**Better Explained**
Record date when a positive symptom first reached at least a 3: ☐ "Ever since I can recall" ☐ Date of onset ___/___Month/ Year	Record most recent date when a positive symptom currently rated 3-6 experienced an increase by at least one rating point:Date of worsening ___/___Month/Year	Check all that apply: ☐ $\geq$ 1h/d, $\geq$ 4d/wk ☐ $\geq$ several minutes/d, $\geq$1x/mo ☐ $\geq$ 1x/wk ☐ none of above	Symptoms are better explained by another Axis I or II disorder. Check one: ☐ Likely ☐ Not likely

P. 4. PERCEPTUAL ABNORMALITIES/HALLUCINATIONS

The following questions probe for both hallucinations and nonpsychotic perceptual abnormalities. They are rated on the SOPS P4 Scale at the end of the queries.

PERCEPTUAL DISTORTIONS, ILLUSIONS, HALLUCINATIONS

Inquiry:

1. **Do you ever feel that your mind is playing tricks on you?** N NI Y **(Record Qualifiers)**

QUALIFIERS: For all "Y" responses, record:

- Description-Onset-Duration-Frequency
- Degree of Distress: What is this experience like for you? (Does it bother you?)
- Degree of interference with life: Do you ever act on this experience? Does having the experience ever cause you to do anything differently?
- Degree of Conviction/Meaning: How do you account for this experience? Do you ever feel that it could just be in your head? Do you think this is real?

____

____

____

____

AUDITORY DISTORTIONS, ILLUSIONS, HALLUCINATIONS

Inquiry:

1. **Do you ever feel that your ears are playing tricks on you?** N NI Y **(Record Qualifiers)**
2. **Have you been feeling more sensitive to sounds?** Have sounds seemed different? Louder or softer? N NI Y **(Record Qualifiers)**
3. **Do you ever hear unusual sounds like banging, clicking, hissing, clapping, ringing in your ears?** N NI Y **(Record Qualifiers)**
4. **Do you ever think you hear sounds and then realize that there is probably nothing there?** N NI Y **(Record Qualifiers)**

5. **Do you ever hear your own thoughts as if they are being spoken outside your head?** N NI Y (Record Qualifiers)
6. **Do you ever hear a voice that others don't seem to or can't hear?** Does it sound clearly like a voice speaking to you as I am now? Could it be your own thoughts or is it clearly a voice speaking out loud? N NI Y (Record Qualifiers)

____
____
____
____
____
____
____
____

VISUAL DISTORTIONS, ILLUSIONS, HALLUCINATIONS

Inquiry:

1. **Do you ever feel your eyes are playing tricks on you?** N NI Y (Record Qualifiers)
2. **Do you seem to feel more sensitive to light or do things that you see ever appear different in color, brightness, or dullness; or have they changed in some other way?** N NI Y (Record Qualifiers)
3. **Have you ever seen unusual things like flashes, flames, vague figures, or shadows out of the corner of your eye?** N NI Y (Record Qualifiers)
4. **Do you ever think you see people, animals, or things, but then realize they may not really be there?** N NI Y (Record Qualifiers)
5. **Do you ever see things that others can't or don't seem to see?** N NI Y (Record Qualifiers)

QUALIFIERS: For all "Y" responses, record:

- Description-Onset-Duration-Frequency
- Degree of Distress: What is this experience like for you? (Does it bother you?)
- Degree of interference with life: Do you ever act on this experience? Does having the experience ever cause you to do anything differently?
- Degree of Conviction/Meaning: How do you account for this experience? Do you ever feel that it could just be in your head? Do you think this is real?

SOMATIC DISTORTIONS, ILLUSIONS, HALLUCINATIONS

Inquiry:

1. **Have you noticed any unusual bodily sensations such as tingling, pulling, pressure, aches, burning, cold, numbness, vibrations, electricity, or pain?** **N NI Y (Record Qualifiers)**

OLFACTORY AND GUSTATORY DISTORTIONS, ILLUSIONS, HALLUCINATIONS

Inquiry:

1. **Do you ever smell or taste things that other people don't notice?** **N NI Y (Record Qualifiers)**

QUALIFIERS: For all "Y" responses, record:

- Description-Onset-Duration-Frequency
- Degree of Distress: What is this experience like for you? (Does it bother you?)
- Degree of interference with life: Do you ever act on this experience? Does having the experience ever cause you to do anything differently?
- Degree of Conviction/Meaning: How do you account for this experience? Do you ever feel that it could just be in your head? Do you think this is real?

P. 4. DESCRIPTION: PERCEPTUAL ABNORMALITIES/ HALLUCINATIONS

a. Unusual perceptual experiences. Heightened or dulled perceptions, vivid sensory experiences, distortions, illusions.
b. Pseudo-hallucinations or hallucinations into which the subject has insight (i.e., is aware of their abnormal nature).
c. Occasional frank hallucinations that may minimally influence thinking or behavior.

Anchors in each scale are intended to provide guidelines and examples of signs for every symptom observed. It is not necessary to meet every criterion in any one anchor to assign a particular rating. Basis for ratings includes both interviewer observations and patient reports.

PERCEPTUAL ABNORMALITIES/HALLUCINATIONS **Severity Scale (circle one)**

0 Absent	1 Questionably Present	2 Mild	3 Moderate	4 Moderately Severe	5 Severe but Not Psychotic	6 Severe and Psychotic
	Minor, but noticeable perceptual sensitivity (e.g., heightened, dulled, distorted, etc.).	Unformed perceptual experiences/ changes that are noticed but not considered to be significant.	Recurrent, unformed, images (e.g., shadows, trails, sounds, etc.), illusions, or persistent perceptual distortions that are puzzling and experienced as unusual.	Illusions or momentary formed hallucinations that are ultimately recognized as unreal yet can be distracting, curious, unsettling. May affect functioning.	Hallucinations experienced as external to self though skepticism can be induced by others. Mesmerizing, distressing. Affects daily functioning.	Hallucinations perceived as real and distinct from the person's thoughts. Skepticism cannot be induced. Captures attention, frightening. Interferes persistently with thinking, feeling, social relations, and/or behavior.

Rating based on:

For Symptoms Rated at Level 3 or Higher			
Symptom Onset	**Symptom Worsening**	**Symptom Frequency**	**Better Explained**
Record date when a positive symptom first reached at least a 3: ☐ "Ever since I can recall" ☐ Date of onset ___/___Month/Year	Record most recent date when a positive symptom currently rated 3-6 experienced an increase by at least one rating point: Date of worsening ___/___Month/Year	Check all that apply: ☐ ≥ 1h/d, ≥ 4d/wk ☐ ≥ several minutes/d, ≥1x/mo ☐ ≥ 1x/wk ☐ none of above	Symptoms are better explained by another Axis I or II disorder. Check one: ☐ Likely ☐ Not likely

P. 5. DISORGANIZED COMMUNICATION

The following questions probe for thought disorder and other difficulties in thinking as reflected in speech. They are rated on the SOPS P5 Scale.

Note: Basis for rating includes: Verbal communication and coherence during the interview as well as reports of problems with speech.

COMMUNICATION DIFFICULTIES

Inquiry:

1. **Do people ever tell you that they can't understand you? Do people ever seem to have difficulty understanding you?** N NI Y (Record Qualifiers)
2. **Are you aware of any ongoing difficulties getting your point across, such as finding yourself rambling or going off track when you talk?** N NI Y (Record Qualifiers)
3. **Do you ever completely lose your train of thought or speech, like suddenly blanking out?** N NI Y (Record Qualifiers)

QUALIFIERS: For all "Y" responses, record:

- Description-Onset-Duration-Frequency
- Degree of Distress: What is this experience like for you? (Does it bother you?)
- Degree of interference with life: Do you ever act on this experience? Does having the experience ever cause you to do anything differently?
- Degree of Conviction/Meaning: How do you account for this experience? Do you ever feel that it could just be in your head? Do you think this is real?

P. 5. DESCRIPTION: DISORGANIZED COMMUNICATION

a. Odd speech. Vague, metaphorical, overelaborate, stereotyped.
b. Confused, muddled, racing or slowed-down speech, using the wrong words, talking about things irrelevant to context or going off track.
c. Speech is circumstantial, tangential, or paralogical. There is some difficulty in directing sentences toward a goal.
d. Loosening or paralysis (blocking) of associations may be present and make speech hard to follow or unintelligible.

Anchors in each scale are intended to provide guidelines and examples of signs for every symptom observed. It is not necessary to meet every criterion in any one anchor to assign a particular rating. Basis for ratings includes both interviewer observations and patient reports.

DISORGANIZED COMMUNICATION **Severity Scale (circle one)**

0 Absent	1 Questionably Present	2 Mild	3 Moderate	4 Moderately Severe	5 Severe but Not Psychotic	6 Severe and Psychotic
	Occasional word or phrase doesn't make sense.	Speech that is slightly vague, muddled, overelaborate, or stereotyped.	Incorrect words, irrelevant topics. Goes off track, but redirects on own.	Speech is circumstantial (i.e., eventually getting to the point). Difficulty directing sentences toward a goal. Sudden pauses. Can be redirected with occasional questions and structuring.	Speech tangential (i.e., never getting to the point). Some loosening of associations or blocking. Can reorient briefly with frequent prompts or questions.	Communication persistently loose, irrelevant, or blocked and unintelligible when under minimal pressure or when the content of the communication is complex. Not responsive to structuring of the interview.

Rating based on:____

For Symptoms Rated at Level 3 or Higher			
Symptom Onset	**Symptom Worsening**	**Symptom Frequency**	**Better Explained**
Record date when a positive symptom first reached at least a 3: ☐ "Ever since I can recall" ☐ Date of onset ___/___Month/Year	Record most recent date when a positive symptom currently rated 3-6 experienced an increase by at least one rating point: Date of worsening ___/___Month/Year	Check all that apply: ☐ ≥ 1h/d, ≥ 4d/wk ☐ ≥ several minutes/d, ≥1x/mo ☐ ≥ 1x/wk ☐ none of above	Symptoms are better explained by another Axis I or II disorder. Check one: ☐ Likely ☐ Not likely

N. NEGATIVE SYMPTOMS

N. 1. SOCIAL ANHEDONIA

Inquiry:

1. **Do you usually prefer to be alone or with others?** (If prefers to be alone, specify reason.) Social apathy? Ill at ease with others? Anxiety? Other? **Record Response**
2. **What do you usually do with your free time?** Would you be more social if you had the opportunity? **Record Response**
3. **How often do you spend time with friends outside of school/work?** Who are your three closest friends? What sorts of activities do you do together? **Record Response**
4. **Who tends to initiate social contact, you or others?** **Record Response**
5. **How often do you spend time with family members?** What do you do with them? **Record Response**

For all responses, record: description, onset, duration, and change over time.

____

____

N. 1. DESCRIPTION: SOCIAL ANHEDONIA

a. Lack of close friends or confidants other than first-degree relatives.
b. Prefers to spend time alone, although participates in social functions when required. Does not initiate contact.
c. Passively goes along with most social activities but in a disinterested or mechanical way. Tends to recede into the background.

Anchors in each scale are intended to provide guidelines and examples of signs for every symptom observed. It is not necessary to meet every criterion in any one anchor to assign a particular rating. Basis for ratings includes both interviewer observations and patient reports.

SOCIAL ANHEDONIA OR WITHDRAWAL **Negative Symptom Scale**

0 Absent	1 Questionably Present	2 Mild	3 Moderate	4 Moderately Severe	5 Severe	6 Extreme
	Slightly socially awkward but socially active.	Ill at ease with others. Only mildly interested in social situations but socially present.	Participates socially only reluctantly due to disinterest. Passively goes along with social activities.	Few friends outside of extended family. Socially apathetic. Minimal social participation.	Significant difficulties with relationships or no close friends. Prefers to be alone. Spends most time alone or with first-degree relatives.	No friends. Prefers being alone.

Rating based on:____

____

____

Symptom Onset (for symptoms rated at a level 3 or higher)
Record date when the earliest symptom first occurred: ☐ Entire lifetime or "ever since I can remember" ☐ Cannot be determined ☐ Date of onset ________________/_______ Month Year

N. 2. AVOLITION

Inquiry:

1. **Do you find that you have trouble getting motivated to do things?**	N	NI	Y	**(Record Response)**
2. **Are you having a harder time getting normal daily activities done? Sometimes? Always? Does prodding work? Sometimes? Never?**	N	NI	Y	**(Record Response)**
3. **Do you find that people have to push you to get things done?** Have you stopped doing anything that you usually do?	N	NI	Y	**(Record Response)**

For all responses, record: description, onset, duration, and change over time.

____

____

____

____

____

N. 2. DESCRIPTION: AVOLITION

a. Impairment in the initiation, persistence, and control of goal-directed activities.
b. Low drive, energy, or productivity.

Anchors in each scale are intended to provide guidelines and examples of signs for every symptom observed. It is not necessary to meet every criterion in any one anchor to assign a particular rating. Basis for ratings includes both interviewer observations and patient reports.

AVOLITION **Negative Symptom Scale**

0 Absent	1 Questionably Present	2 Mild	3 Moderate	4 Moderately Severe	5 Severe	6 Extreme
	Focus on goal-directed activities but less than what would be considered average.	Low drive or energy level. Simple tasks require effort or take longer than what would be considered normal. Productivity is considered average or is within normal limits.	Low levels of motivation to participate in goal-directed activities. Impairment in task initiation and/or persistence. Initiation or task completion requires some prodding.	Minimal levels of motivation to participate in or complete goal-directed activities. Prodding needed regularly.	Lack of drive/ energy results in a significantly low level of achievement. Most goal-directed activities relinquished. Prodding is needed all of the time, but may not be successful.	Prodding unsuccessful. Not participating in virtually any goal-directed activities.

Rating based on:____

____

____

____

Symptom Onset (for symptoms rated at a level 3 or higher)
Record date when the earliest symptom first occurred: ☐ Entire lifetime or "ever since I can remember" ☐ Cannot be determined ☐ Date of onset ______________/_______ Month Year

N. 3. EXPRESSION OF EMOTION

Inquiry:

1. **Has anyone pointed out to you that you are less emotional or connected to people than you used to be?** **N NI Y (Record Response)**

For all responses, record: description, onset, duration, and change over time.

Note: Basis for rating includes: Observed flattened affect as well as reports of decreased expression of emotion.

____

____

____

N. 3. DESCRIPTION: EXPRESSION OF EMOTION

a. Flat, constricted, diminished emotional responsiveness as characterized by a decrease in expression, modulation of feelings (e.g., monotone speech) and communication gestures (e.g., dull appearance).
b. Lack of spontaneity and flow of conversation. Reduction in the normal flow of communication. Conversation shows little initiative. Patient's answers tend to be brief and unembellished, requiring direct and sustained questions by interviewer.
c. Poor rapport. Lack of interpersonal empathy, openness in conversation, sense of closeness, interest, or involvement with the interviewer. This is evidenced by interpersonal distancing and reduced verbal and non-verbal communication.

Anchors in each scale are intended to provide guidelines and examples of signs for every symptom observed. It is not necessary to meet every criterion in any one anchor to assign a particular rating. Basis for ratings includes both interviewer observations and patient reports.

EXPRESSION OF EMOTION **Negative Symptom Scale**

0 Absent	1 Questionably Present	2 Mild	3 Moderate	4 Moderately Severe	5 Severe	6 Extreme
	Emotional responsiveness slightly delayed or blunted.	Conversation lacks liveliness, feels stilted.	Emotional expression minimal at times but maintains flow of conversation.	Difficulty in sustaining conversation. Speech mostly monotone. Minimal interpersonal empathy. May avoid eye contact.	Starting and maintaining conversation requires direct and sustained questioning by the interviewer. Affect constricted. Total lack of gestures.	Flat affect, monotone speech. Unable to become involved with interviewer or maintain conversation despite active questioning by the interviewer.

Rating based on:____

____

____

____

Symptom Onset (for symptoms rated at a level 3 or higher)
Record date when the earliest symptom first occurred: ☐ Entire lifetime or "ever since I can remember" ☐ Cannot be determined ☐ Date of onset ____________/______ Month Year

N. 4. EXPERIENCE OF EMOTIONS AND SELF

Inquiry:

1. **Do your emotions feel less strong in general than they used to?** Do you ever feel numb? **N NI Y (Record Response)**
2. **Do you find yourself having a harder time distinguishing different emotions/feelings?** **N NI Y (Record Response)**
3. **Are you feeling emotionally flat?** **N NI Y (Record Response)**
4. **Do you ever feel a loss of sense of self or feel disconnected from yourself or your life?** Like a spectator in your own life? **N NI Y (Record Response)**

For all responses, record: description, onset, duration, and change over time.

____

____

N. 4. DESCRIPTION: EXPERIENCE OF EMOTIONS AND SELF

a. Emotional experiences and feelings less recognizable and genuine, appropriate.
b. Sense of distance when talking to others, not feeling rapport with others.
c. Emotions disappearing, difficulty feeling happy or sad.
d. Sense of having no feelings: Anhedonia, apathy, loss of interest, boredom.
e. Feeling profoundly changed, unreal, or strange.
f. Feeling depersonalized, at a distance from self.
g. Loss of sense of self.

Anchors in each scale are intended to provide guidelines and examples of signs for every symptom observed. It is not necessary to meet every criterion in any one anchor to assign a particular rating. Basis for ratings includes both interviewer observations and patient reports.

EXPERIENCE OF EMOTIONS AND SELF **Negative Symptom Scale**

0 Absent	1 Questionably Present	2 Mild	3 Moderate	4 Moderately Severe	5 Severe	6 Extreme
	Feeling distant from others. Everyday feelings muted.	Lack of strong emotions or clearly defined feelings.	Emotions feel like they are blunted or not easily distinguishable.	Sense of deadness, flatness, or undifferentiated aversive tension. Difficulty feeling emotions, even emotional extremes, (e.g., happy/sad).	Feeling a loss of sense of self. Feeling depersonalized, unreal, or strange. May feel disconnected from body, from world, from time. No feelings most of the time.	Feeling profoundly changed and possibly alien to self. No feelings.

Rating based on:____

Symptom Onset (for symptoms rated at a level 3 or higher)
Record date when the earliest symptom first occurred: ☐ Entire lifetime or "ever since I can remember" ☐ Cannot be determined ☐ Date of onset __________/______ Month Year

N.5. IDEATIONAL RICHNESS

Inquiry:

1. **Do you sometimes find it hard to understand what people are trying to tell you because you don't understand what they mean?** **N NI Y (Record Response)**
2. **Do people more and more use words you don't understand?** **N NI Y (Record Response)**

For all responses, record: description, onset, duration, and change over time

ABSTRACTION QUESTIONS:

Similarities— How are the following alike?
A ball and an orange?__________
An apple and a banana?__________
A painting and a poem?__________
Air and water?__________

Proverbs — "What does this saying mean?"
a. Don't judge a book by its cover.__________
b. Don't count your chickens before they hatch.__________

N. 5. DESCRIPTION: IDEATIONAL RICHNESS

a. Unable to make sense of familiar phrases or to grasp the "gist" of a conversation or to follow everyday discourse.
b. Stereotyped verbal content. Decreased fluidity, spontaneity, and flexibility of thinking, as evidenced in repetitious, or simple thought content. Some rigidity in attitudes or beliefs. Does not consider alternative positions or has difficulty shifting from one idea to another.
c. Simple words and sentence structure; paucity of dependent clauses or modifications (adjectives/adverbs).

d. Difficulty in abstract thinking. Impairment in the use of the abstract-symbolic mode of thinking, as evidenced by difficulty in classification, forming generalizations, and proceeding beyond concrete or egocentric thinking in problem-solving tasks; often utilizes a concrete mode.

Anchors in each scale are intended to provide guidelines and examples of signs for every symptom observed. It is not necessary to meet every criterion in any one anchor to assign a particular rating. Basis for ratings includes both interviewer observations and patient reports.

IDEATIONAL RICHNESS Negative Symptom Scale

0 Absent	1 Questionably Present	2 Mild	3 Moderate	4 Moderately Severe	5 Severe	6 Extreme
	Some conversational awkwardness.	Trouble grasping nuances of conversation. Diminished conversational give and take.	Correctly interprets most similarities and proverbs. Uses few modifiers (adjectives and adverbs). May miss some abstract comments.	At times misses the "gist" of reasonably uncomplicated conversation. Verbal content may be repetitious and perseverative. Uses simple words and sentence structure without many modifiers. Misses or interprets many similarities and proverbs concretely.	Able to follow and answer simple statements and questions, but has difficulty independently articulating thoughts and experiences. Verbal content restricted and stereotyped. Verbal expression limited to simple, brief sentences. May be unable to interpret most similarities and proverbs.	Unable, at times, to follow any conversation no matter how simple. Verbal content and expression mostly limited to single words and yes/no responses.

Rating based on: ____________________

____

____

____

Symptom Onset (for symptoms rated at a level 3 or higher)
Record date when the earliest symptom first occurred: ☐ Entire lifetime or "ever since I can remember" ☐ Cannot be determined ☐ Date of onset ________/____ Month Year

N. 6. OCCUPATIONAL FUNCTIONING

Inquiry:

1. **Does your work take more effort than it used to?** **N NI Y (Record Response)**
2. **Are you having a hard time getting your work done?** **N NI Y (Record Response)**
3. **Have you been doing worse in school or at work?** Have you been put on probation or otherwise given notice due to poor performance? Are you failing any classes or considering dropping out of school? Have you ever been "let go" from a job, or are otherwise having trouble keeping a job? **N NI Y (Record Response)**

For all responses, record: description, onset, duration, and change over time.

____

____

____

____

N. 6. DESCRIPTION: OCCUPATIONAL FUNCTIONING

a. Difficulty performing role functions (e.g., wage earner, student, homemaker) that were previously performed without problems.
b. Having difficulty in productive, instrumental relationships with colleagues at work or school.

Anchors in each scale are intended to provide guidelines and examples of signs for every symptom observed. It is not necessary to meet every criterion in any one anchor to assign a particular rating. Basis for ratings includes both interviewer observations and patient reports.

OCCUPATIONAL FUNCTIONING **Negative Symptom Scale**

0 Absent	1 Questionably Present	2 Mild	3 Moderate	4 Moderately Severe	5 Severe	6 Extreme
	More than average effort and focus required to maintain usual level of performance at work, school.	Difficulty in functioning at work or school that is becoming evident to others.	Definite problems in accomplishing work tasks or a drop in Grade Point Average.	Failing one or more courses. Receiving notice or being on probation at work.	Suspended, failing out of school, or other significant interference with completing requirements. Problematic absence from work. Unable to work with others.	Failed or left school, left employment or was fired.

Rating based on: ____

____

____

____

____

Symptom Onset (for symptoms rated at a level 3 or higher)
Record date when the earliest symptom first occurred: ☐ Entire lifetime or "ever since I can remember" ☐ Cannot be determined ☐ Date of onset ________________/_______ Month Year

D. DISORGANIZATION SYMPTOMS

D. 1. ODD BEHAVIOR OR APPEARANCE

Inquiry:

1. What kinds of activities do you like to do?				**(Record Response)**
2. Do you have any hobbies, special interests, or collections?	**N**	**NI**	**Y**	**(Record Response)**
3. Do you think others ever say that your interests are unusual or that you are eccentric?	**N**	**NI**	**Y**	**(Record Response)**

For all responses, record: description, onset, duration, and change over time.

Note: Basis for rating includes: Interviewer observations of unusual or eccentric appearance as well as reports of eccentric, unusual, or bizarre behavior or appearance.

____

____

____

____

D. 1. DESCRIPTION: ODD BEHAVIOR OR APPEARANCE

a. Behavior or appearance that is odd, eccentric, peculiar, disorganized, or bizarre.
b. Appears preoccupied with and/or interactive with own thoughts.
c. Inappropriate affect.

Anchors in each scale are intended to provide guidelines and examples of signs for every symptom observed. It is not necessary to meet every criterion in any one anchor to assign a particular rating. Basis for ratings includes both interviewer observations and patient reports.

ODD BEHAVIOR/APPEARANCE **Disorganization Symptom Scale**

0 Absent	1 Questionably Present	2 Mild	3 Moderate	4 Moderately Severe	5 Severe	6 Extreme
	Questionably unusual appearance, behavior.	Behavior or appearance that appears minimally unusual or odd.	Odd, unusual behavior, interests, appearance, hobbies, or preoccupations that are likely to be considered outside of cultural norms. May exhibit some inappropriate behavior.	Behavior or appearance, that is unconventional by most standards. May appear distracted by apparent internal stimuli. May seem disengaging or off-putting.	Highly unconventional strange behavior or appearance. May, at times, seem preoccupied by apparent internal stimuli. May provide noncontextual responses, or exhibit inappropriate affect. May be ostracized by peers.	Grossly bizarre appearance or behavior (e.g., collecting garbage, talking to self in public). Disconnection of affect and speech.

Rating based on: ______________________________

____

____

____

____

Symptom Onset (for symptoms rated at a level 3 or higher)
Record date when the earliest symptom first occurred: ☐ Entire lifetime or "ever since I can remember" ☐ Cannot be determined ☐ Date of onset ________________/________ Month Year

D. 2. BIZARRE THINKING

Inquiry:

1. **Do people ever say your ideas are unusual or that the way you think is strange or illogical?** **N NI Y (Record Response)**

For all responses, record: description, onset, duration, and change over time.

Note: Basis for rating includes: Observations of unusual or bizarre thinking as well as reports of unusual or bizarre thinking.

D.2. DESCRIPTION: BIZARRE THINKING

a. Thinking characterized by strange, fantastic, or bizarre ideas that are distorted, illogical, or patently absurd.

Anchors in each scale are intended to provide guidelines and examples of signs for every symptom observed. It is not necessary to meet every criterion in any one anchor to assign a particular rating. Basis for ratings includes both interviewer observations and patient reports.

BIZARRE THINKING **Disorganization Symptom Scale**

0 Absent	1 Questionably Present	2 Mild	3 Moderate	4 Moderately Severe	5 Severe	6 Extreme
	"Quirky" ideas that are easily abandoned.	Unusual ideas, illogical or distorted thinking.	Unusual ideas, illogical or distorted thoughts that are held as a belief or philosophical system within the realm of subcultural variation.	Unusual ideas or illogical thinking that is embraced but which violates the boundary of most conventional religious or philosophical thoughts.	Strange ideas that are difficult to understand.	Thoughts that are fantastic, patently absurd, fragmented, and impossible to understand.

Rating based on:

Symptom Onset (for symptoms rated at a level 3 or higher)
Record date when the earliest symptom first occurred: ☐ Entire lifetime or "ever since I can remember"] ☐ Cannot be determined ☐ Date of onset ________/____ Month Year

D. 3. TROUBLE WITH FOCUS AND ATTENTION

Inquiry:

1. **Have you had difficulty concentrating or being able to focus on a task?** Reading? Listening? Is this getting worse than it was before? **N NI Y (Record Response)**
2. **Are you easily distracted? Easily confused by noises, by other people speaking? Is this getting worse? Have you had trouble remembering things?** **N NI Y (Record Response)**

For all responses, record: description, onset, duration, and change over time.

Note: Basis for rating includes: Interviewer observations or patient reports of trouble with focus and attention.

____

____

____

____

____

D. 3. DESCRIPTION: TROUBLE WITH FOCUS AND ATTENTION

a. Failure in focused alertness, manifested by poor concentration, distractibility from internal and external stimuli.
b. Difficulty in harnessing, sustaining, or shifting focus to new stimuli.
c. Trouble with short-term memory including holding conversation in memory.

Anchors are intended to provide guidelines and examples of signs for every symptom observed. It is not necessary to meet every criterion in any one anchor to assign a particular rating. Basis for ratings includes interviewer observations and patient reports.

TROUBLE WITH FOCUS AND ATTENTION **Disorganization Symptom Scale**

0 Absent	1 Questionably Present	2 Mild	3 Moderate	4 Moderately Severe	5 Severe	6 Extreme
	Lapses of focus under pressure.	Inattention to everyday tasks or conversations.	Problems maintaining focus and attention. Difficulty keeping up with conversations.	Distracted and often loses track of conversations.	Can maintain attention and remain in focus only with outside structure or support.	Unable to maintain attention even with external refocusing.

Rating based on: ____

____

____

____

____

Symptom Onset (for symptoms rated at a level 3 or higher)
Record date when the earliest symptom first occurred: ☐ Entire lifetime or "ever since I can remember" ☐ Cannot be determined ☐ Date of onset ________________/_______ Month Year

D. 4. IMPAIRMENT IN PERSONAL HYGIENE

Inquiry:

1. **Are you less interested in keeping clean or dressing well?** **N NI Y (Record Response)**
2. **How often do you shower?** **(Record Response)**
3. **When is the last time you went shopping for new clothes?** **(Record Response)**

For all responses, record: description, onset, duration, and change over time.

____

____

____

____

____

____

D. 4. DESCRIPTION: IMPAIRMENT IN PERSONAL HYGIENE

a. Impairment in personal hygiene and grooming. Self-neglect.

Anchors in each scale are intended to provide guidelines and examples of signs for every symptom observed. It is not necessary to meet every criterion in any one anchor to assign a particular rating. Basis for ratings includes both interviewer observations and patient reports.

IMPAIRMENT IN PERSONAL HYGIENE **Disorganization Symptom Scale**

0 Absent	1 Questionably Present	2 Mild	3 Moderate	4 Moderately Severe	5 Severe	6 Extreme
	Low attention to personal hygiene, but still concerned with appearances.	Low attention to personal hygiene and little concern with physical or social appearance, but still within bounds of convention and/or subculture.	Indifference to conventional and/or subcultural conventions of dress and social cues.	Neglect of social or subcultural norms of hygiene.	Does not bathe regularly. Clothes unkempt, unchanged, unwashed. May have developed an odor.	Poorly groomed and appears not to care or even notice. No bathing and has developed an odor. Inattentive to social cues and unresponsive even when confronted.

Rating based on: ______________________________

____

____

____

____

____

Symptom Onset (for symptoms rated at a level 3 or higher)
Record date when the earliest symptom first occurred: ☐ Entire lifetime or "ever since I can remember" ☐ Cannot be determined ☐ Date of onset ________________/_______ Month Year

G. GENERAL SYMPTOMS

G. 1. SLEEP DISTURBANCE

Inquiry:

1. **How have you been sleeping recently?** What kinds of difficulty have you been having with your sleep? (include time to bed, to sleep, and to awake, hours of sleep in a 24-hour period, difficulty falling asleep, early awakening, day/night reversal). **(Record Response)**
2. **Do you find yourself tired during the day?** Is your problem with sleeping making it difficult to get through your day? Do you have trouble waking up? **N NI Y (Record Response)**

For all responses, record: description, onset, duration, and change over time.

Note: Basis for rating includes: Hypersomnia and hyposomnia.

____

____

____

____

G.1. DESCRIPTION: SLEEP DISTURBANCE

a. Having difficulty falling asleep.
b. Waking earlier than desired and not able to fall back asleep.
c. Daytime fatigue and sleeping during the day.
d. Day/night reversal.
e. Hypersomnia.

Anchors in each scale are intended to provide guidelines and examples of signs for every symptom observed. It is not necessary to meet every criterion in any one anchor to assign a particular rating. Basis for ratings includes both interviewer observations and patient reports.

SLEEP DISTURBANCE **General Symptom Scale**

0 Absent	1 Questionably Present	2 Mild	3 Moderate	4 Moderately Severe	5 Severe	6 Extreme
	Restless sleep.	Some mild difficulty falling asleep or getting back to sleep.	Daytime fatigue resulting from difficulty falling asleep at night or early awakening. Sleeping more than considered average.	Sleep pattern significantly disrupted and has intruded on other aspects of functioning (e.g., trouble getting up for school or work). Difficult to awaken for appointments. Spending a large part of the day asleep.	Significant difficulty falling asleep or awakening early on most nights. May have day/night reversal. Usually not getting to scheduled activities at all.	Unable to sleep at all for over 48 hours.

Rating based on: ______________________________

____

____

____

Symptom Onset (for symptoms rated at a level 3 or higher)
Record date when the earliest symptom first occurred: ☐ Entire lifetime or "ever since I can remember" ☐ Cannot be determined ☐ Date of onset ________/________ Month Year

G.2. DYSPHORIC MOOD

Inquiry:

1. **What has your mood been like recently?** **(Record Response)**
2. **Do you ever generally just feel unhappy for any length of time?** **N NI Y (Record Response)**
3. **Have you ever been depressed?** Do you find yourself crying a lot? Do you feel sad/bad/worthless/hopeless? Has your mood affected your appetite? Your sleep? Your ability to work? **N NI Y (Record Response)**
4. **Have you had thoughts of harming yourself or ending your life?** Have you ever attempted suicide? **N NI Y (Record Response)**

5. **Have you had thoughts of harming anyone else?** **N NI Y (Record Response)**
6. **Do you find yourself feeling irritable a lot of the time?** Do you get angry often? Do you ever hit anyone or anything? **N NI Y (Record Response)**
7. **Have you felt more nervous, anxious lately? Has it been hard for you to relax?** **N NI Y (Record Response)**

For all responses, record: description, onset, duration, and change over time.

____

____

G. 2. DESCRIPTION: DYSPHORIC MOOD

a. Diminished interest in pleasurable activities.
b. Sleeping problems.
c. Poor or increased appetite
d. Feelings of loss of energy.
e. Difficulty concentrating.
f. Suicidal thoughts.
g. Feelings of worthlessness and/or guilt.

a. Anxiety, panic, multiple fears and phobias.
b. Irritability, hostility, rage.
c. Restlessness, agitation, tension.
d. Unstable mood.

Anchors in each scale are intended to provide guidelines and examples of signs for every symptom observed. It is not necessary to meet every criterion in any one anchor to assign a particular rating. Basis for ratings includes both interviewer observations and patient reports.

DYSPHORIC MOOD **General Symptom Scale**

0 Absent	1 Questionably Present	2 Mild	3 Moderate	4 Moderately Severe	5 Severe	6 Extreme
	Feeling "down" or edgy often.	Occasional unstable and/or unpredictable periods of sad, bad, or dark feelings that may be a mixture of depression, irritability, or anxiety.	Feelings like the "blues" or other anxieties or discontents have "settled in."	Recurrent periods of sadness, irritability, or depression.	Persistent unpleasant mixtures of depression, irritability, or anxiety. Avoidance behaviors such as substance use or sleep.	Painfully unpleasant mixtures of depression, irritability, or anxiety that may trigger highly destructive behaviors like suicide attempts or self-mutilation.

Rating based on:____

____

____

Symptom Onset (for symptoms rated at a level 3 or higher)
Record date when the earliest symptom first occurred: ☐ Entire lifetime or "ever since I can remember" ☐ Cannot be determined ☐ Date of onset ________________/_______ Month Year

G. 3. MOTOR DISTURBANCES

Inquiry:

1. **Have you noticed any clumsiness, awkwardness, or lack of coordination in your movements?** **N NI Y (Record Response)**

For all responses, record: description, onset, duration, and change over time.

____

____

____

____

____

G. 3. DESCRIPTION: MOTOR DISTURBANCES

a. Reported or observed clumsiness, lack of coordination, difficulty performing activities that were performed without problems in the past.
b. The development of a new movement such as a nervous habit, stereotypes, characteristic ways of doing something, posture, or copying other peoples' movements (echopraxia).
c. Motor blockages (catatonia).
d. Loss of automatic skills.
e. Compulsive motor rituals.
f. Dyskinetic movements of head, face, extremities.

Anchors in each scale are intended to provide guidelines and examples of signs for every symptom observed. It is not necessary to meet every criterion in any one anchor to assign a particular rating. Basis for ratings includes both interviewer observations and patient reports.

MOTOR DISTURBANCES **General Symptom Scale**

0 Absent	1 Questionably Present	2 Mild	3 Moderate	4 Moderately Severe	5 Severe	6 Extreme
	Awkward.	Reported or observed clumsiness.	Poor coordination. Difficulty performing fine motor movements.	Stereotyped, often inappropriate movements.	Nervous habits, tics, grimacing. Posturing. Compulsive motor rituals.	Loss of natural movements. Motor blockages. Echopraxia. Dyskinesia.

Rating based on: ____

____

____

____

____

Symptom Onset (for symptoms rated at a level 3 or higher)
Record date when the earliest symptom first occurred: ☐ Entire lifetime or "ever since I can remember" ☐ Cannot be determined ☐ Date of onset ________________/_______ Month Year

G. 4. IMPAIRED TOLERANCE TO NORMAL STRESS

Inquiry:

1. **Are you feeling more tired or stressed than the average person at the end of a usual day?** **N NI Y (Record Response)**
2. **Do you get thrown off by unexpected things that happen to you during the day?** **N NI Y (Record Response)**
3. **Are you finding that you are feeling challenged or overwhelmed by some of your daily activities?** Are you avoiding any of your daily activities? **N NI Y (Record Response)**
4. **Are you finding yourself too stressed, disorganized, or drained of energy and motivation to cope with daily activities?** **N NI Y (Record Response)**

For all responses, record: description, onset, duration, and change over time.

G.4. DESCRIPTION: IMPAIRED TOLERANCE TO NORMAL STRESS

a. Avoids or exhausted by stressful situations that were previously dealt with easily.
b. Marked symptoms of anxiety or avoidance in response to everyday stressors.
c. Increasingly affected by experiences that were easily handled in the past. More difficulty habituating.

Anchors in each scale are intended to provide guidelines and examples of signs for every symptom observed. It is not necessary to meet every criterion in any one anchor to assign a particular rating. Basis for ratings includes both interviewer observations and patient reports.

IMPAIRED TOLERANCE TO NORMAL STRESS **General Symptom Scale**

0 Absent	1 Questionably Present	2 Mild	3 Moderate	4 Moderately Severe	5 Severe	6 Extreme
	Tired or stressed at end of usual day.	Daily stress brings on symptoms of anxiety beyond what might be expected.	Thrown off by unexpected happenings in the usual day.	Increasingly "challenged" by daily experiences.	Avoids or is overwhelmed by stressful situations that arise during day.	Disorganization, panic, apathy, or withdrawal in response to everyday stress.

Symptom Onset (for symptoms rated at a level 3 or higher)

Record date when the earliest symptom first occurred:

- ☐ Entire lifetime or "ever since I can remember"
- ☐ Cannot be determined
- ☐ Date of onset ________/____
  Month Year

GLOBAL ASSESSMENT OF FUNCTIONING

GAF-M: When scoring consider psychological, social, and occupational functioning on a hypothetical continuum of mental health/illness. Do not include impairment in functioning due to physical health (or environmental) limitations.

NO SYMPTOMS: 100–91
Superior functioning in a wide range of activities Life's problems never seem to get out of hand Sought out by others because of his or her many positive qualities *A person doing exceptionally well in all areas of life = rating 95–100* *A person doing exceptionally well with minimal stress in one area of life = rating 91–94*
ABSENT OR MINIMAL SYMPTOMS: 90–81
Minimal or absent symptoms (e.g., mild anxiety before an examination) Good functioning in all areas and satisfied with life Interested and involved in a wide range of activities Socially effective No more than everyday problems or concerns (e.g., an occasional argument with family members) *A person with no symptoms or everyday problems = rating 88–90* *A person with minimal symptoms or everyday problems = rating 84–87* *A person with minimal symptoms and everyday problems = rating 81–83*
SOME TRANSIENT SYMPTOMS: 80–71
Mild symptoms are present, but they are transient and expectable reactions to psychosocial stressors (e.g., difficulty concentrating after family argument) Slight impairment in social, work, or school functioning (e.g., temporarily falling behind in school or work) *A person with EITHER mild symptom(s) OR mild impairment in social, work, or school functioning = rating 78–80* *A person with mild impairment in more than 1 area of social, work, or school functioning = rating 74–77* *A person with BOTH mild symptoms AND slight impairment in social, work, and school functioning = rating 71–73*
SOME PERSISTENT MILD SYMPTOMS: 70–61
Mild symptoms are present that are NOT just expectable reactions to psychosocial stressors (e.g., mild or lessened depression and/or mild insomnia) Some persistent difficulty in social, occupational, or school functioning (e.g., occasional truancy, theft within the family, or repeated falling behind in school or work) BUT has some meaningful interpersonal relationships *A person with EITHER mild persistent symptoms OR mild difficulty in social, work, or school functioning = rating 68–70* *A person with mild persistent difficulty in more than 1 area of social, work, or school functioning = rating 64–67* *A person with BOTH mild persistent symptoms AND some difficulty in social, work, and school functioning = rating 61–63*

MODERATE SYMPTOMS: 60–51
Moderate symptoms (e.g., frequent, depressed mood and insomnia and/or moderate ruminating and obsessing; or occasional anxiety attacks; or flat affect and circumstantial speech; or eating problems and below minimum safe weight without depression) Moderate difficulty in social, work, or school functioning (e.g., few friends or conflicts with co-workers) *A person with EITHER moderate symptoms OR moderate difficulty in social, work, or school functioning = rating 58–60* *A person with moderate difficulty in more than 1 area of social, work, or school functioning = rating 54–57* *A person with BOTH moderate symptoms AND moderate difficulty in social, work, and school functioning = rating 51–53*
SOME SERIOUS SYMPTOMS OR IMPAIRMENT IN FUNCTIONING: 50–31
Serious impairment with work, school, or housework if a housewife/househusband (e.g., unable to keep a job or stay in school, or failing school, or unable to care for family and house) Frequent problems with the law (e.g., frequent shoplifting, arrests) or occasional combative behavior Serious impairment in relationships with friends (e.g., very few or no friends, or avoids what friends s/he has) Serious impairment in relationships with family (e.g., frequent fights with family and/or neglects family or has no home) Serious impairment in judgment (including inability to make decisions, confusion, disorientation) Serious impairment in thinking (including constant preoccupation with thoughts, distorted body image, paranoia) Serious impairment in mood (including constant depressed mood plus helplessness and hopelessness, or agitation, or manic mood) Serious impairment due to anxiety (panic attacks, overwhelming anxiety) Other symptoms: some hallucinations, delusions, or severe obsessional rituals Passive suicidal ideation *A person with 1 area of disturbance = rating 48–50* *A person with 2 areas of disturbance = rating 44–47* *A person with 3 areas of disturbance = rating 41–43* *A person with 4 areas of disturbance = rating 38–40* *A person with 5 areas of disturbance = rating 34–37* *A person with 6 areas of disturbance = rating 31–33*
INABILITY TO FUNCTION IN ALMOST ALL AREAS: 30–21
Suicidal preoccupation or frank suicidal ideation with preparation OR behavior considerably influenced by delusions or hallucinations OR serious impairment in communication (sometimes incoherent, acts grossly inappropriately, or profound stuporous depression) Serious impairment with work, school, or housework if a housewife/househusband (e.g., unable to keep a job or stay in school, or failing school, or unable to care for family and house) Frequent problems with the law (e.g., frequent shoplifting, arrests) or occasional combative behavior

Serious impairment in relationships with friends (e.g., very few or no friends, or avoids what friends s/he has) Serious impairment in relationships with family (e.g., frequent fights with family and/or neglects family or has no home) Serious impairment in judgment (including inability to make decisions, confusion, disorientation) Serious impairment in thinking (including constant preoccupation with thoughts, distorted body image, paranoia) Serious impairment in mood (including constant depressed mood plus helplessness and hopelessness, or agitation, or manic mood) Serious impairment due to anxiety (panic attacks, overwhelming anxiety) Other symptoms: some hallucinations, delusions, or severe obsessional rituals Passive suicidal ideation *A person with any 1 of the first 3 (unique) criteria = rating 21* *OR a person with 7 of the combined criteria = rating 28–30* *A person with 8-9 of the combined criteria = rating 24–27* *A person with 10 of the combined criteria = rating 20–23*
IN SOME DANGER OF HURTING SELF OR OTHERS: 20–11
Suicide attempts without clear expectation of death (e.g., mild overdose or scratching wrists with people around) Some severe violence or self-mutilating behaviors Severe manic excitement, or severe agitation and impulsivity Occasionally fails to maintain minimal personal hygiene (e.g., diarrhea due to laxatives, or smearing feces) Urgent/emergency admission to the present psychiatric hospital In physical danger due to medical problems (e.g., severe anorexia or bulimia and some spontaneous vomiting or extensive laxative/diuretic/diet pill use, but without serious heart or kidney problems or severe dehydration and disorientation) *A person with 1–2 of the 6 areas of disturbance in this category = rating 18–20* *A person with 3–4 of the 6 areas of disturbance in this category = rating 14–17* *A person with 5–6 of the 6 areas of disturbance in this category = rating 11–13*
IN PERSISTENT DANGER OF SEVERELY HURTING SELF OR OTHERS: 10–1
Serious suicidal act with clear expectation of death (e.g., stabbing, shooting, hanging, or serious overdose, with no one present) Frequent severe violence or self-mutilation Extreme manic excitement, or extreme agitation and impulsivity (e.g., wild screaming and ripping the stuffing out of a bed mattress) Persistent inability to maintain minimal personal hygiene Urgent/emergency admission to present psychiatric hospital In acute, severe danger due to medical problems (e.g., severe anorexia or bulimia with heart/kidney problems, or spontaneous vomiting WHENEVER food is ingested, or severe depression with out-of-control diabetes) *A person with 1–2 of the 6 areas of disturbance in this category = rating 8–10* *A person with 3–4 of the 6 areas of disturbance in this category = rating –7* *A person with 5–6 of the 6 areas of disturbance in this category = rating 1–3*

Adapted from: Hall, R. (1995). Global assessment of functioning: A modified scale, *Psychosomatics*, *36*, 267–275.

Current Score: ___________ **Highest Score in Past Year:**___________

SCHIZOTYPAL PERSONALITY DISORDER CRITERIA

Genetic Risk and Deterioration Prodromal State—Genetic risk involves meeting DSM-IV criteria for Schizotypal Personality Disorder (see below) and/or having a first-degree relative with a psychotic disorder (see p. 7).

DSM IV - Schizotypal Personality Disorder:
A pervasive pattern of social and interpersonal deficits marked by acute discomfort with, and reduced capacity for close relationships as well as by cognitive or perceptual distortions and eccentricities of behavior. Onset can be traced back at least to adolescence or early adulthood. In persons under age 18 years, features must have been present for at least 1 year.

Current Schizotypal Personality Disorder as Indicated by Five (or more) of the Following:

DSM IV - Schizotypal Personality Disorder Criteria - Rated based on responses to the interview.	Yes	No
a. Ideas of reference (excluding delusions of reference)		
b. Odd beliefs or magical thinking that influences behavior and is inconsistent with subculture norms (e.g., superstitiousness, belief in clairvoyance, telepathy, or "sixth sense"; in children and adolescents, bizarre fantasies or preoccupations)		
c. Unusual perceptual experiences, including bodily illusions		
d. Odd thinking and speech (e.g., vague, metaphorical, over-elaborate, stereotyped)		
e. Suspiciousness or paranoid ideation		
f. Inappropriate or constricted affect		
g. Behavior or appearance that is odd, eccentric, or peculiar		
h. Lack of close friends or confidants other than first-degree relatives		
i. Excessive social anxiety that does not diminish with familiarity and tends to be associated with paranoid fears rather than negative judgments about self		
Does the patient meet criteria for DSM IV— Schizotypal Personality Disorder?		

SUMMARY OF SIPS DATA

Positive Symptom Scale

0 Absent	1 Questionably Present	2 Mild	3 Moderate	4 Moderately Severe	5 Severe but Not Psychotic	6 Severe and Psychotic

Positive Symptoms

P1. Unusual Thought Content/Delusional Ideas	0	1	2	3	4	5	6
P2. Suspiciousness/Persecutory Ideas	0	1	2	3	4	5	6
P3. Grandiosity	0	1	2	3	4	5	6
P4. Perceptual Abnormalities/Hallucinations	0	1	2	3	4	5	6
P5. Disorganized Communication	0	1	2	3	4	5	6

Negative, Disorganization, General Symptom Scale

0 Absent	1 Questionably Present	2 Mild	3 Moderate	4 Moderately Severe	5 Severe	6 Extreme

Negative Symptoms

N1. Social Anhedonia	0	1	2	3	4	5	6
N2. Avolition	0	1	2	3	4	5	6
N3. Expression of Emotion	0	1	2	3	4	5	6
N4. Experience of Emotions and Self	0	1	2	3	4	5	6
N5. Ideational Richness	0	1	2	3	4	5	6
N6. Occupational Functioning	0	1	2	3	4	5	6

Disorganization Symptoms

D1. Odd Behavior or Appearance	0	1	2	3	4	5	6
D2. Bizarre Thinking	0	1	2	3	4	5	6
D3. Trouble with Focus and Attention	0	1	2	3	4	5	6
D4. Personal Hygiene	0	1	2	3	4	5	6

General Symptoms

G1. Sleep Disturbance	0	1	2	3	4	5	6
G2. Dysphoric Mood	0	1	2	3	4	5	6
G3. Motor Disturbances	0	1	2	3	4	5	6
G4. Impaired Tolerance to Normal Stress	0	1	2	3	4	5	6

GAF (p. 37) Current______ Highest in Past Year______
Schizotypal Personality Disorder (p. 38) yes______ no______
Family History of Psychotic Illness (p. 7) yes______ no______

SUMMARY OF SIPS SYNDROME CRITERIA

I. Rule out Current and Past Psychosis: Presence of Psychotic Syndrome (POPS)

Psychotic Syndrome		**Yes**	**No**
A.	Are any of the SOPS P1–P5 Scales scored 6, or have they ever been?		
B.	If Yes to A, are the symptoms seriously disorganizing or dangerous, or were they ever?		
C.	If Yes to A, did the symptoms occur for at least one hour per day at an average frequency of four days per week over one month?		

If Yes to A and B or A and C, the subject meets criteria for current psychosis.
Note: Date when criteria first achieved (mm/dd/yy): ____________________

II. Rule in Psychosis-Risk Syndrome: Criteria of Psychosis-risk Syndromes (COPS 3.0)

A. Brief Intermittent Psychotic Symptom Psychosis-Risk Syndrome		**Yes**	**No**
1.	Are any of the SOPS P1–P5 Scales scored 6?		
2.	If Yes to 1, have the symptoms reached a psychotic level of intensity in the past three months?		
3.	If Yes to 1 and 2, are the symptoms currently present for at least several minutes per day at a frequency of at least once per month?		
4.	Are all otherwise qualifying symptoms better explained by another DSM-IV disorder (Axis I or II)?		

If 1–3 are Yes and 4 is No, the subject meets criteria for Brief Intermittent Psychotic Syndrome.
Note: Date when criteria first achieved (mm/dd/yy): ____________________

B. Attenuated Positive Symptom Psychosis-Risk Syndrome		**Yes**	**No**
1.	Are any of the SOPS P1–P5 Scales scored 3–5?		
2.	If Yes to 1, have any of these symptoms begun within the past year or do any currently rate one or more scale points higher compared to 12 months ago?		
3.	If Yes to 1 and 2, have the symptoms occurred at an average frequency of at least once per week in the past month?		
4.	Are all otherwise qualifying symptoms better explained by another DSM—IV disorder (Axis 1 or 2)?		

If 1–3 are Yes and 4 is a No, the subject meets criteria for Attenuated Positive Symptom Prodromal Syndrome.
Note: Date when criteria first achieved (mm/dd/yy): ____________________

C. Genetic Risk and Deterioration Psychosis-Risk Syndrome		Yes	No
1.	The patient meets criteria for Schizotypal Personality Disorder.		
2.	The patient has a first-degree relative with a psychotic disorder.		
3.	The patient is experiencing at least a 30% drop in GAF score over the last month as compared to 12 months ago.		

If any of the following conditions are met:

1. 1 and 3
2. 2 and 3
3. 1 and 2 and 3

The subject meets criteria for Genetic Risk and Deterioration Psychosis-Risk Syndrome.
Note: Date when criteria first achieved (mm/dd/yy): ____________________

Please check yes or no.

__ **No**	__ **Yes**	**Psychotic Syndrome**
__ **No**	__ **Yes**	**Brief Intermittent Psychotic Symptom Psychosis-Risk Syndrome**
__ **No**	__ **Yes**	**Attenuated Positive Symptom Psychosis-Risk Syndrome**
__ **No**	__ **Yes**	**Genetic Risk and Deterioration Psychosis-Risk Syndrome**
__ **No**	__ **Yes**	**Other DSM-IV Disorders**
		Axis I ______________, ______________, ______________
		Axis II ______________, ______________, ______________

Appendix C

Informed Consent

Consent for Participation in a Research Project
(Parent/Guardian of Minor)
Yale University School of Medicine

INVITATION TO PARTICIPATE AND DESCRIPTION OF PROJECT

Title of Study: Delaying or Preventing Psychosis: A Clinical Trial of Olanzapine in Persons Prodromal to Psychosis

You (your child) are invited to participate in this research study designed to determine if certain kinds of early treatment reduce the risk for serious mental illness. Psychosis is a type of serious mental illness in which people can hear or see things that others cannot hear or see, hold strong beliefs about things that are not really true, take poor care of themselves, and/or have trouble making sense. People may experience milder forms of these symptoms such as having unusual perceptions, feeling suspicious of others sometimes without true cause, having trouble organizing their speech such that others have trouble following what they are saying, or feeling flat, unreal, unmotivated, and unrelated like they have lost their emotions. Sometimes these milder experiences don't go away or get worse and lead to psychosis, which is serious. Other times these milder symptoms go away with time or treatment. At the present time, we do not know what makes the difference between these symptoms' going away, staying, or getting worse. Understanding these outcomes better is one of the purposes of this study.

Psychotic experiences can be treated effectively with counseling and what are called antipsychotic medications. Preliminary studies suggest that these types of medications can also be used to treat milder forms of psychotic experiences as well. Therefore, in this study we plan to test whether an antipsychotic medication called olanzapine is better than placebo (sugar pill) in reducing symptoms and possibly preventing the symptoms from coming back, getting worse, or leading to psychosis.

You have been invited to participate because you have been struggling with symptoms and problems that may be milder forms of psychotic experiences. Please note that we do not know this for sure. What you are going through may be temporary and/or unrelated to psychosis. We want to find out by inviting you to participate in this study where we can follow you with clinical tests over time.

While the goal of this study is to help you feel better and more in control of your life, it is possible that you will feel worse, especially if you are receiving placebo. This is a risk of your being in the study. You may also feel worse due to the side effects of olanzapine. If you are in the study and your condition gets worse it will be noticed rapidly because you will be making regular visits to the doctor. If this happens, you will get more treatment; for example, more study drug and/or counseling.

There may be risks from your participation in this study. Olanzapine has to date been taken by about 6,900 (study) patients and has been used in the treatment of over three and one half million people.

(Next is detailed all common and uncommon side effects of the drug.)

Your participation in this study may involve receiving treatment that is not necessary or specific to your problem. Furthermore, participation in this study may lead you to worry unnecessarily about having or developing a more serious problem when in fact that might not happen. We hope that by paying careful attention to you and your clinical symptoms over time, the study doctors will help you to manage such anxieties by giving you the benefit of reassurance if things are well and help if things are not.

This study may provide some benefit to you. You will receive family and/or individual counseling on a regular basis and for any crisis. You may receive information about your health from any physical examinations and laboratory tests that are done in this study. Furthermore, the availability of careful and responsive ongoing clinical testing is one of the benefits of this study. The study offers a system of careful monitoring that could spot troubles rapidly and start appropriate treatments early. If you develop problems they may be identified and evaluated much faster since you will be making regular visits to the doctor.

Index

Note: Page numbers followed by *f* and *t* denote figures and tables, respectively.

Printed in the USA/Agawam, MA
June 8, 2015

616455.042